Preparing for the Future of Combat Casualty Care

Opportunities to Refine the Military Health System's Alignment with the National Defense Strategy

BRENT THOMAS

Prepared for the Office of the Secretary of Defense
Approved for public release; distribution unlimited

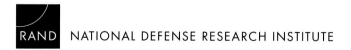

NATIONAL DEFENSE RESEARCH INSTITUTE

For more information on this publication, visit www.rand.org/t/RRA713-1

Library of Congress Cataloging-in-Publication Data is available for this publication.
ISBN: 978-1-9774-0686-6

Published by the RAND Corporation, Santa Monica, Calif.
© Copyright 2021 RAND Corporation
RAND® is a registered trademark.

Cover photo: Sarayuth Pinthong, Air Force/Department of Defense

Support RAND
Make a tax-deductible charitable contribution at
www.rand.org/giving/contribute

www.rand.org

Preface

The Military Health System (MHS) comprises a global network of treatment facilities and medical providers. During day-to-day operations, health care coverage under the MHS benefit extends to more than 9 million beneficiaries, including active-duty and reserve-component service members, military retirees, and their families. In addition to providing health care during peacetime, the MHS also offers medical care to troops injured in combat.

Although the MHS has proved capable in treating wounded service members in recent conflict environments, the 2018 National Defense Strategy (NDS) highlights how future combat operations may be distinctly different from those of the past few decades. For example, potential adversaries are investing in long-range, high-precision missile systems. With these capabilities, an adversary might choose to direct strikes against operational infrastructure, such as runways and fuel reserves. Loss of these assets can significantly degrade U.S. combat capabilities.

Furthermore, with large-scale missile strikes, casualty streams are likely to be quite significant at operating locations across the combat theater. High casualty volume can sorely tax the capability, capacity, and throughput of deployed medical care. But challenges to medical support resulting from adversary action could be even more direct. For example, it is dangerous to evacuate patients during active combat, and treatment facilities close to conflict operations could, themselves, be at risk of an adversary strike.

In parallel, Congress has directed the MHS to realign some of its responsibilities to improve the overall efficiency of its day-to-day health care operations. These reforms have required significant institutional time and energy, but they have been transformative for the MHS. Transitioning governance of military treatment facilities to the Defense Health Agency has required numerous changes to the way the MHS operates, including a restructuring of management functions, the development of a new electronic health record system, a reassessment of MTF infrastructure requirements, and an evaluation of reposturing options for medical staffing billets, all of which are now the responsibility of operational military forces.

The analysis in this report assesses the potential ramifications of this confluence of an evolving threat environment and the recent congressionally mandated reforms to the MHS. This report highlights specific challenges driven by the future operating environments outlined in the NDS and the associated requirements for combat casualty care. Given the increased focus on efficiencies in the structure and governance of the MHS, the findings and recommendations presented here underscore the potential ramifications for combat medical care in scenarios with far greater numbers of combat casualties than the United States has seen in recent history.

The objective of this research was to identify medical support domains in which MHS capabilities could benefit from closer alignment with potential future threats. In exploring an array of possible challenges that clinicians, medical logisticians, and the medical supply industrial base might need to grapple with in supporting future combat operations, it also suggests a range of mitigation strategies for the MHS to pursue to close capability gaps. These mitigations support an agile force reconstitution, resilient logistics, and robust sustainment, enhancing the MHS mission set and increasing support of the warfighter both at home and in combat.

This report should be of particular interest to military medical providers and planners, as well as operators, logisticians, and contingency operations planners across the U.S. Department of Defense. Shared supply chains, common manufacturers, and the U.S. military's potential need to rely on civilian health care facilities mean that this study's findings could also be of interest to the industrial base for medical supplies and public health planners in the United States and abroad.

The research reported here was completed in November 2020 and underwent security review with the sponsor and the Defense Office of Prepublication and Security Review before public release.

This research was sponsored by the Office of the Secretary of Defense and conducted within the Forces and Resources Policy Center of the RAND National Security Research Division (NSRD), which operates the National Defense Research Institute (NDRI), a federally funded research and development center sponsored by the Office of the Secretary of Defense, the Joint Staff, the Unified Combatant Commands, the Navy, the Marine Corps, the defense agencies, and the defense intelligence enterprise.

For more information on the RAND Forces and Resources Policy Center, see www.rand.org/nsrd/frp or contact the director (contact information is provided on the webpage).

Contents

Figures and Tables

Figures

Tables

Summary

The National Defense Strategy (NDS), published by the Office of the Secretary of Defense roughly every four years, outlines the direction that the U.S. Department of Defense (DoD) will take to prepare for the global security environment in which it will operate.[1] The NDS, itself, is informed by the executive branch's national security plans and concerns, which are captured in a separate document known as the U.S. National Security Strategy. As such, the NDS informs investments to modernize the force, adapt the U.S. global force posture, and amendments to military policy and strategy to keep them aligned with future challenges.

The Growing Risk of High-Intensity Conflict

The 2018 NDS notes that such potential adversaries as China, Russia, Iran, and North Korea have been investing in long-range, precision missile systems. In response, DoD senior leaders have shifted their thinking about requirements for future combat to ensure the resilience and, ultimately, success of U.S. forces in high-intensity conflict environments. One key element of that planning falls to the Military Health System (MHS), which must ensure that combat casualty care

---

[1] U.S. Department of Defense, *Summary of the 2018 National Defense Strategy of the United States of America: Sharpening the American Military's Competitive Edge*, Washington, D.C., 2018.

can surmount challenges to medical support that may arise in this future battlespace.

Improving Efficiencies in the Military Health System

In recent years, Congress has directed the MHS to realign some of the responsibilities among its entities. The intent of the realignment was to improve the overall efficiency of day-to-day health care operations across the system. These reforms have been transformative for the MHS, and they have required significant institutional time and energy. For example, transitioning governance of military treatment facilities (MTFs) to the Defense Health Agency (DHA) has entailed not only a restructuring of management functions but also the development of a new electronic health record system, a reassessment of MTF infrastructure requirements, and an evaluation of reposturing options that could move medical staffing billets out of the MHS and into operational military forces.[2]

Additionally, Congress has directed that DHA's responsibilities include "coordinating with the military departments to ensure that the staffing at the military medical treatment facilities supports readiness requirements" for military operations.[3] With its intense focus on transitioning day-to-day health care operations to DHA, the MHS could benefit from a fresh external examination of what these "readiness requirements" might entail. Namely, it could prove informative to examine readiness through the question of what the MHS might

---

[2]   These changes were enacted through the National Defense Authorization Acts (NDAAs) for fiscal years 2017 and 2019. For more on the shift to DHA in managing the care of service members, their dependents, and military retirees across the network of MTFs, see MHS, "MHS Transformation," webpage, undated, and U.S. Code, Title 10, Section 1073c, Administration of Defense Health Agency and Military Medical Treatment Facilities.

The MTFs' transition to DHA was ongoing as of this writing. Cuts to MHS medical billets could exceed 17,000 positions. See Tom Philpott, "More Than 17,000 Uniformed Medical Jobs Eyed for Elimination," *Military.com*, January 10, 2019.

[3]   Public Law 116–92, National Defense Authorization Act for Fiscal Year 2020, December 20, 2019, Section 712, Support by Military Health System of Medical Requirements of Combatant Commands, para. (b)(1).

need to be ready for in providing medical support in future military operations.

Aligning MHS Operations with Evolving Threats

This report presents an analysis of the potential ramifications of this confluence of an evolving threat environment and the ongoing reforms to MHS operations. It highlights specific challenges and effects on requirements for combat casualty care. Given that the structure and governance of the MHS has changed under recent NDAAs to focus on identifying efficiencies, the report underscores the risks of under-preparing for potentially vastly increased numbers of casualties than U.S. forces have seen in recent contingencies. The findings raise important questions about the degree to which future operational requirements would stress existing military medical capabilities.

The objective of this study was to identify where MHS capabilities might benefit from closer alignment with the threats that U.S. forces could face in future conflicts. The findings are intended to help clinicians, medical logisticians, and the industrial base for medical supplies prepare for the challenges of supporting future combat operations, and this report suggests a range of mitigation strategies that the MHS could pursue to help close capability gaps in these areas. However, this report is merely a first step in addressing these issues. A more-detailed study is warranted to quantify gaps and to recommend priorities for implementing mitigation options to support an agile force, resilient logistics, robust sustainment, enhanced MHS mission sets, and increased support to the warfighter both at home and in combat.

Developing a clear vision to prepare the medical community for future conflicts can be a daunting prospect. Planning for combat medical support sits at a difficult nexus. It involves integrating a diverse set of stakeholder equities, drawing on military intelligence estimates to evaluate adversary threats, interacting with medical providers to establish a list of required clinical capabilities, and drawing insights from medical logisticians to gain a broader view of where medical practitioners will require sustainment and support. Developing a common plan that integrates insights from each stakeholder group will be essential to success in combat.

Research Approach

To help the MHS identify opportunities to better prepare for the challenges highlighted by the NDS, this report draws on open-source literature exploring how future conflict environments might differ from those of recent decades. It also identifies possible stress points in the network of care that could inhibit the treatment of combat casualties or complicate patient movement from the point of injury to a nearby field hospital and onward to hospitals in the United States (for those requiring more-comprehensive medical care). The analysis was structured around seven research questions:

- How has DoD's picture of global threats evolved over the past decade?
- How might weapons on the future battlefield drive different compositions of casualty streams, in terms of both casualty numbers and the distribution of injuries?
- Are expeditionary MTFs prepared to receive those casualties and offer care at a level that wounded service members have received in recent decades?
- Given the changing global threat picture that the NDS outlines, are the services able to rapidly establish an expeditionary network of care to receive combat casualties?
- Is the current MHS posture of medical logistics and sustainment optimized for the likely requirements of a future fight?
- Does the NDS mission of homeland defense introduce additional stressors that the MHS should consider?
- Could the stressors of a future fight ripple into the industrial base that supports the MHS in caring for combat casualties?

Although this is not an exhaustive set of relevant questions, the answers highlight a range of opportunities for the MHS to mitigate risk and close potential capability gaps. This survey of challenges is intended to provide an overview candidate problem sets and areas where further analysis could inform future investment in research and development, training, materiel solutions, and other capabilities to improve medical outcomes in future combat operations.

It is important to note that this report does not explicitly address the implications for the MHS in the event of chemical, biological, radiological, or nuclear (CBRN) attacks on a future battlefield. One reason is that the intelligence assessments for these attack modes are rarely discussed in the open literature. That said, it is reasonable to assume CBRN weapon employment would drive a requirement for medical resources far larger than what would be expected in the wake of a conventional attack.

For example, a CBRN attack could accompany a conventional missile strike, so the baseline patient load could include casualties seeking treatment for trauma injuries. But a medical facility receiving CBRN casualties should be prepared to decontaminate patients before they are admitted for treatment. Similarly, if a biological vector is suspected, a mechanism for isolating the infected should be employed to ensure that the spread of the biological agent is restricted. By imposing these additional requirements, a medical facility's patient treatment rate would be expected to decline at a time when there is elevated demand for facility space, caregiver time, and medical supplies.

The following recommendations for the MHS are extracted from themes in the literature and the analytic results presented in this report.

Recommendations

Prepare Combat Casualty Care for a Rapidly Evolving Set of Global Threats

Rather than organizing, training, and equipping the medical force for a fight that resembles recent military operations in Iraq and Afghanistan, the MHS should consider how evolving threat conditions might change the requirements for medical support in a future fight. For example, adversaries are heavily investing in advanced missile systems, a combat capability that stands to generate more (and more-severe) casualties than U.S. forces have encountered in a century.

Forecast Likely Requirements for Care on the Future Battlefield

The MHS evolved agile, efficient networks of deployed medical personnel, facilities, and supply chains capable of quickly stabilizing, treating, and evacuating wounded service members from the Iraq and Afghanistan theaters. It saw tremendous success in treating patients injured in the line of duty and limiting loss of life. However, that posture of medical support has evolved on the predicates of relatively light patient loads and air superiority for U.S. forces to safely evacuate patients to higher echelons of care as needed. As projected in the 2018 NDS, in future large-scale combat operations, these assumptions might no longer consistently apply.

Adversary weapon systems, such as ballistic and cruise missiles, could yield large numbers of blast casualties. Weaponeering analysis suggests that the types of injuries to be expected in these blast events will be similar to those encountered in recent conflicts, but their numbers could be significantly greater. In tandem, by targeting the infrastructure that supports military mobility, an adversary can readily degrade U.S freedom of movement. In future combat operations, large streams of trauma patients and degraded evacuation availability could tax or overwhelm the capability, capacity, and throughput of deployed military medical care.

Enhance Treatment Options at and Near the Point of Injury

In preparing for future combat operations with constraints on the capability of available medical personnel to offer high-quality care to the wounded, the capacity of field hospitals to treat and hold large numbers of combat casualties, and the ability to expedite patient throughput at expeditionary MTFs, the MHS has several mitigations to choose from, and it will most likely want to adopt portfolios of mitigations to address potential gaps in all three areas (capability, capacity, and throughput). For example, better training for first responders (the injured service member, who could administer self-help first aid, and nearby service members) could improve medical capability; augmenting modular MTFs, especially by expanding critical care wards, can help increase patient holding capacity where it is most needed; and pairing resilient resupply mechanisms with triage strategies specific to mass trauma events can accelerate patient throughput.

Evaluate the Benefits of an Expanded Posture of Prepositioned Medical Assets

Given that the 2018 NDS speaks to the potential for a rapid onset of hostilities in the future combat environment, it is important to ensure that critical medical assets are close at hand, and that the U.S. military's network of expeditionary MTFs is in place before the first wave of combat casualties requires treatment.

Cold War–era planners recognized this possibility as well, and a robust network of prepositioned materiel was established in Europe to ensure that needed capability could be set up in the field quickly. Given that robust prepositioning postures have languished in the intervening years, medical planners will likely need to consider a range of options to invigorate the U.S. military's global medical warehousing network. In pursuing this mitigation approach, the MHS has to address several questions, including what to store, where to warehouse it, how to maintain it, and how to move it to likely points of end use. Additional assessments will be key to determining the cost-effectiveness of sustaining the network, how to track effectiveness and speed; and which assets will be available and how they will be transported to their intended points of end use.

Consider Options to Improve the Resilience of Medical Logistics and Sustainment Capabilities

Medical logistics plays an important role in ensuring access to medical support. The special handling and maintenance requirements of many types of stored medical materiel mean there is a need for periodic inspection, repair, and replacement. The MHS has a range of manpower options to support these operations, but it must carefully balance the cost-saving potential of civilian and contract labor against requirements to deploy military personnel in these roles who are able provide broader support for contingency operations.

Where there are gaps in asset maintenance and sustainment support, the MHS could benefit from expanded agreements with partner nations. Moreover, all medical logistics support is predicated on reliable and enduring situational awareness of what assets are where, at what levels, and in what condition. To sustain that awareness in a contested environment during combat, the MHS might need to consider ways to enhance the resilience of key data systems and communication links.

Prepare for Homeland Support and Homeland Defense Missions

The 2018 NDS emphasizes not only the growing potential for conflict overseas but also the heightened need for military support closer to home. Thus, the MHS should consider how adversary threats may drive the need for medical support in the Arctic, for example, and the ramifications for the care of trauma patients in that environment. Because large numbers of casualties could return to CONUS, the MHS would benefit from a clearer map of the rights and authorities involved in managing the flow of patients both within the MHS network and to civilian care facilities.

Build Resilience into the Industrial Base for Medical Supplies

In delivering medical support to large numbers of combat casualties, the MHS may see effects that ripple farther upstream in the medical supply chains, where surge demand could outstrip the capacity of the medical supply industrial base. In their day-to-day support to the MHS, manufacturers can generally meet contracted demands for medical supplies. However, given how the industrial base has achieved significant cost-effectiveness through advances in production efficiencies, access to some supplies could be far more constrained under the surge-demand conditions of a large-scale contingency. This may prove especially true for low-cost goods, such as saline and generic pharmaceuticals, for which supply chains can be long and the industrial base may lack meaningful surge production capacity.

The MHS should consider options to diversify its partnerships with the industrial base—possibly in concert with interagency partners—and invest in enhanced manufacturing practices to more quickly meet surge-demand signals. It could also help international partners enhance their quality-control processes to better align with U.S. Food and Drug Administration practices and regulations. In so doing, the MHS can help mitigate the risk of supply shortages while promoting flexibility in industrial supply chain operations.

Conclusions

Individual mitigations can have significant value in improving casualty care quality and access. However, no single solution appears to be a "silver bullet" that will broadly improve the performance of expeditionary medical care in the conflict scenarios posited by the 2018 NDS. Consequently, it is important for the MHS to develop portfolios of options and to assess each portfolio with respect to its overall cost and performance. For example, which mitigation portfolios would be most cost-effective in improving return-to-duty rates? Do they combine materiel and training solutions, such as investing in a broader network of medical WRM storage sites and expanding training for first responders? Or do they involve a shift in current policy, with increased investment in partner-nation medical support capabilities and enhancements to the industrial base for medical supplies? Clear answers to these questions were not immediately apparent from a review of recent literature. Consequently, as the MHS evaluates these considerations, it will be better positioned to inform decisionmakers and stakeholders of key cost points and where forecasted capabilities will offer maximum benefit.

The NDS has shone a light on an array of considerations for the MHS and projects a future threat environment that is starkly different from the U.S. military's experiences in recent contingencies. This has significantly changed the operational view for front-line combat units and the capabilities they need to prepare to employ against a future adversary. To sustain the warfighter's combat capability, combat service support functions, such as medical, are facing an equally daunting paradigm shift. Careful reflection on the challenges outlined in the 2018 NDS reveals a range of opportunities to improve the capability of the MHS in a future fight. With the objective of building a more agile force, the MHS has numerous options to bring resilient logistics and robust sustainment to its enhanced posture and to optimize its support for the warfighter both at home and in combat.

Acknowledgments

For their support to the ideas found in this report, I would like to extend my warmest thanks to a range of sponsors, collaborators, and colleagues. No hard work is accomplished alone, and no good idea occurs in a vacuum.

RAND first began exploring issues related to combat casualty care in the era of rapidly evolving threats under the guidance of Air Force medical leadership, including Lt Gen (ret.) Thomas Travis, Lt Gen (ret.) Mark Ediger, and Lt Gen Dorothy Hogg. I am indebted to their insights and guidance, and for setting RAND down this course.

Members of the medical leadership at U.S. Pacific Air Forces were also instrumental in shaping and informing the insights in this report. I extend countless thanks, in particular, to Brig Gen Paul Friedrichs, Brig Gen Rob Marks, and Col Joseph Anderson for their support and helpful framing.

Several colleagues at U.S. Central Command were pivotal in sharing insights regarding the potential challenges for medical logistics in a future fight. I would like to thank MAJ Andrew Wilson, LCDR Nicole Dutton, and Jim Sjovall for all that they dedicated to exploring this space.

In terms of the ramifications of partner-nation medical support, this report would have been wholly incomplete without insights from colleagues at U.S. European Command. COL (ret.) Ron Smith, CAPT Mark Kobelja, COL Sean Keenan, COL Jay Baker, and Lt Col Mike Kersten shared their discerning vision for the future of medical support.

With respect to discussions on industrial base capabilities, I extend my enduring gratitude to the Joint Trauma System (JTS) and especially to Col Stacey Shackelford and COL Jennifer Gurney. Opportunities to engage with the JTS always lead to reflections informed by a great depth of expertise.

Similarly, the exploration of logistics and industrial base capabilities in this report was greatly aided by discussions with Army medical logistics colleagues, including COL Matt Voyles from the Defense Logistics Agency and COL David Sloniker and LTC Autumn Leveridge from the 6th Medical Logistics Management Center.

This report would not have been possible without insights stemming from discussions with colleagues at RAND who also work extensively with the military's health care community. Many thanks to Trupti Brahmbhatt, Kimberly Hepner, Heather Krull, and Tepring Piquado.

RAND's economists also shared key insights to shape the report. Here, I extend my gratitude to Elizabeth Hastings Roer and Grant Johnson.

The dedication and hard work of RAND's Medical Operations in Denied Environments team established the fundamental underpinnings of this study. My humblest thanks to Bradley DeBlois, Beth Grill, Anthony DeCicco, Katherine Hastings, Samantha McBirney, and Katherine Pfrommer.

The clarity and presentation of the narrative were greatly improved by feedback from the document's dedicated review team: Sarah Meadows, Bradley Martin, COL William Fox, and Craig Bond.

Finally, from the RAND management team, I would like to thank John Winkler and Molly McIntosh. Their help in developing the overarching theme for this report was central to its cohesion and clarity, and their support for the work was instrumental in its execution.

Abbreviations

A2AD	anti-access/area denial
AMR	antimicrobial-resistant
CBRN	chemical, biological, radiological, or nuclear
CDO	contested, degraded, or operationally limited
CONUS	continental United States
DCAM	Defense Medical Logistics Standard Support Customer Assistance Module
DHA	Defense Health Agency
DMLSS	Defense Medical Logistics Standard Support Customer
DoD	U.S. Department of Defense
EMEDS	Expeditionary Medical Support
FDA	U.S. Food and Drug Administration
HADR	humanitarian assistance/disaster relief
JMAR	Joint Medical Asset Repository
JMPT	Joint Medical Planning Tool
MEB	Marine expeditionary brigade

MHS	Military Health System
MPTk	Medical Planners' Toolkit
mTBI	mild traumatic brain injury
MTF	military treatment facility
NATO	North Atlantic Treaty Organization
NDAA	National Defense Authorization Act
NDS	National Defense Strategy
OODA	orient, observe, decide, act
PCOF	Patient Condition Occurrence Frequency
POI	point of injury
PRePO	Prepositioning Requirements Planning Optimization
SA	situational awareness
TEWLS	Theater Enterprise-Wide Logistics System
TPFDD	time-phased force and deployment data
TPMRC	theater patient movement requirements center
UAV	unmanned aerial vehicle
WRM	war reserve materiel

CHAPTER ONE

The Challenges of Future Conflict Framed by the National Defense Strategy

The Military Health System (MHS) comprises a global network of treatment facilities and medical providers. In day-to-day operations, health care coverage under the MHS benefit extends to more than 9 million beneficiaries, including active-duty and eligible reserve-component service members, military retirees, and their families. In addition to providing health care during peacetime, the MHS treats service members who are injured during combat.[1]

Several U.S. Department of Defense (DoD) organizations contribute to MHS operations. For example,

- The Office of the Assistant Secretary of Defense for Health Affairs leads the MHS, providing policy and budgeting oversight across the network.
- The Defense Health Agency (DHA), a joint organization founded in 2013, integrates a wide array of functions to manage the joint health enterprise. It oversees health care delivery and maintains medical information systems.
- Military treatment facilities (MTFs) form a network of more than 50 hospitals and almost 400 clinics operated by the U.S. military around the globe.
- The Uniformed Services University of the Health Sciences provides medical education to many military health care providers.

---

[1] For more information on the composition and the MHS and the benefits it offers, refer to Military Health System, homepage, undated.

- The Office of the Joint Staff Surgeon advises the Chairman of the Joint Chiefs of Staff on medical issues and coordinates medical planning across the military's combatant commands.
- The military services manage and deliver medical care to their personnel who are deployed to overseas operations.

In recent years, Congress has directed the MHS to realign some responsibilities among these entities. The intent of the realignment was to improve the overall efficiency of day-to-day health care operations across the system.[2] These changes were enacted through the National Defense Authorization Acts (NDAAs) for fiscal years 2017 and 2019. One key shift was that Congress tasked DHA with managing care for service members, their dependents, and military retirees across the network of MTFs.[3] Prior to the enactment of these NDAAs, the services were responsible for managing MTFs. These reforms have been transformative for the MHS, but they have required significant institutional time and energy. For example, transitioning responsibilities to DHA required not only a restructuring of management functions but also the development of a new electronic health record system, a reassessment of MTF infrastructure requirements, and an evaluation of a possible reposturing of medical staffing billets from the MHS to the operational military forces.[4] The MTFs' transition to DHA was ongoing at the time of this writing.

Additionally, Congress has directed that DHA's responsibilities include "coordinating with the military departments to ensure that the staffing at the military medical treatment facilities supports readiness requirements" for military operations.[5] With its intense focus on transi-

---

[2] See Military Health System, "MHS Transformation," webpage, undated.

[3] U.S. Code, Title 10, Section 1073c, Administration of Defense Health Agency and Military Medical Treatment Facilities.

[4] Cuts to MHS medical billets could exceed 17,000 positions. See Tom Philpott, "More Than 17,000 Uniformed Medical Jobs Eyed for Elimination," *Military.com*, January 10, 2019.

[5] Public Law 116–92, National Defense Authorization Act for Fiscal Year 2020, December 20, 2019, Section 712, Support by Military Health System of Medical Requirements of Combatant Commands, para. (b)(1).

tioning day-to-day health care operations to DHA, the MHS may benefit from a fresh external examination of what these "readiness requirements" might entail. It may prove informative to examine readiness through the question of what the MHS needs to be ready for in terms of providing medical support during future military operations.

Over the past decade, DoD has acknowledged significant changes in the nature of the threats that U.S. forces will face in future combat operations. These shifts in the threat environment have been driving questions about possible challenges to casualty care. This report highlights specific challenges driven by these future operating environments and how they will affect requirements for combat casualty care. Given how the structure and governance of the MHS has changed under recent NDAAs—with a focus on efficiencies—this report also underscores the potential ramifications for combat medical care, particularly where casualties could occur in significantly greater numbers than in recent historical contingencies. These factors raise important questions about the degree to which future operational requirements will stress existing military medical capabilities.

The objective of the analysis in this report was to identify medical support domains where MHS capabilities could benefit from closer alignment against threats to U.S. forces that have been identified in intelligence assessments. By exploring an array of possible challenges that clinicians, medical logisticians, and the industrial base for medical supplies may face in supporting future combat operations, the analysis also suggested a range of mitigation strategies that the MHS could pursue to close capability gaps. This report highlights where more-detailed research is warranted to quantify gaps and recommend priorities for the implementation of mitigation options. Through mitigations that support a more agile force, resilient logistics, and robust sustainment, mission sets across the MHS would be enhanced, ensuring greater support for the warfighter both at home and in combat.

Approach

To help frame where the MHS might find opportunities to better support future combat operations, the analysis presented here drew on open-source literature to explore how future conflict environments might differ from those of recent decades. This was followed by a literature review to identify possible stress points in the network of care that might evolve during the treatment of combat casualties—as patients move from the point of injury (POI) to a nearby field hospital and onward to hospitals in the United States (for those who require more-comprehensive medical care). The analysis was structured around seven research questions:

- How has DoD's picture of global threats evolved over the past decade?
- How might weapons on the future battlefield drive different compositions of casualty streams, in terms of both casualty numbers and the distribution of injuries?
- Are expeditionary MTFs prepared to receive those casualties and offer care at a level that wounded service members have received in recent decades?
- Given the characteristics of the changing global threat picture, are the services able to rapidly establish an expeditionary network of care to receive combat casualties?
- Is the current MHS posture of medical logistics and sustainment optimized for the likely requirements of a future fight?
- Does the special mission of homeland defense introduce additional stressors that the MHS should consider?
- Could the stressors of a future fight ripple into the industrial base that supports the MHS in caring for combat casualties?

Although this set of questions is not an exhaustive catalog, the answers highlight a range of opportunities for the MHS to mitigate risk and close potential capability gaps. This survey of challenges is intended to provide an overview of candidate problem sets and areas where further analysis could inform future investment in research and development, training, materiel solutions, and other capabilities to improve medical outcomes in future combat operations.

To identify relevant literature to address these questions, this study relied on a range of sources: peer-reviewed academic articles, federal government publications, publicly available DoD documents and press releases, media articles, and academic texts collected through searches of the Defense Technical Information Center database,[6] the Web of Science index, and the Nexis Uni database. Supplementing the literature review, subject-matter experts provided additional input and source suggestions.

Although every effort was made to conduct a comprehensive review of relevant policy documents, research on casualty care, MHS and service-level capability data, historical analysis, and other materials, there may have been some limitations to this search tied to the recency of submissions to the respective databases.

The Evolution of the Global Threat Environment

It is useful to begin by examining the changing global threat picture and how U.S. military policy and strategy are responding. For example, as potential adversaries have increased their investment in precision strike capabilities, DoD has taken this shift into account in its planning.

Threats in the Indo-Pacific

In 2011, in an address to the Australian Parliament, President Barack Obama outlined a fundamental shift in U.S. policy in the Indo-Pacific region. As the United States began to draw down its presence in Iraq and Afghanistan, it would begin to rebalance its attention to the Pacific. The purpose of this rebalance, also known as the "pivot to the Pacific," was twofold.

---

[6] For example, this database contains not only publicly available DoD documents but also DoD-funded research, such as RAND reports.

First, the renewed focus on the region would invigorate regional partnerships that had been underserved during extended U.S. combat operations in the Middle East. The goal was to reenergize old alliances and economic ties with such nations as South Korea, Australia, and Japan and to hasten the development of relationships with Indonesia, Thailand, Malaysia, and many others.

Second, the rebalance would foster opportunities to strengthen regional security. Some countries in the Indo-Pacific, including China and North Korea, had been investing in long-range, high-precision weapon programs, including ballistic and cruise missile development.[7] Analysis suggests that the size of China's active-duty force has declined since the mid-1990s, yet its overall military spending and capability have increased significantly, due in part to this modernization and expansion of its ballistic and cruise missile inventories.[8]

With a more manifest demonstration of capability, North Korean military leadership has opted to not only invest in a larger, more capable missile quiver but also to conduct conspicuous tests of its missile platforms as a way of advertising its growing capability on the world stage. Since 2003, North Korea progressively escalated its annual rate of missile launches, which reached a peak in 2017.[9]

Should the United States engage in combat with a nation that has long-range precision missile strike capabilities, these weapons be used against U.S. operating locations from afar and without a direct commitment of the adversary's troops. Consequently, it was thought that this renewed U.S. dedication to its security posture in the Indo-Pacific

---

[7] For discussions of China's ambitions in the open-source literature, see Dennis M. Gormley, Andrew S. Erickson, and Jingdong Yuan, *A Low-Visibility Force Multiplier: Assessing China's Cruise Missile Ambitions*, Washington, D.C., National Defense University Press, 2014, and Eric Heginbotham, Michael Nixon, Forrest E. Morgan, Jacob L. Heim, Jeff Hagen, Sheng Tao Li, Jeffrey Engstrom, Martin C. Libicki, Paul DeLuca, David A. Shlapak, David R. Frelinger, Burgess Laird, Kyle Brady, and Lyle J. Morris, *The U.S.-China Military Scorecard: Forces, Geography and the Evolving Balance of Power, 1996–2017*, Santa Monica, Calif.: RAND Corporation, RR-392-AF, 2015.

[8] Heginbotham et al., 2015.

[9] Center for Strategic and International Studies, "Missiles of North Korea," *Missile Threat*, last updated November 30, 2020c.

would help reduce regional tensions and deter potential adversaries from initiating such a conflict.

Advancing Threats in Europe

As the United States began to rebalance its attention toward the Indo-Pacific, potential adversaries in other regions did not slow their own development of precision missile systems. These growing threats became increasingly pronounced in Europe, where Russia's missile capabilities were becoming a point of concern.

Over the past two decades, Russia has significantly modernized its inventory. A key aspect of its research and development effort has been directed toward enhancing the capability and depth of its cruise missile stockpile.[10] In 2011, Russia's defense minister announced that the country would procure an inventory of missiles with larger payloads and more-advanced guidance systems over the next ten years.[11] In late 2016, intelligence sources reported that the Russian government had moved several Iskander missile systems to the Kaliningrad region. Wedged between NATO members Lithuania and Poland, Kaliningrad provides Russian missiles with a launch point significantly west of the rest of the country, along with an expanded array of potential targets across Europe.[12]

It is worth noting that Russian defense spending has decreased significantly since the dissolution of the Soviet Union in 1991. Although the size of Russia's military and related budget have decreased, the Russian missile inventory has remained well stocked. As a means of projecting military power, a sizable missile arsenal can act as both a cost-effective and credible deterrent and a capable combat platform.[13]

---

[10] Center for Strategic and International Studies, "Missiles of Russia," *Missile Threat*, last updated August 24, 2020b.

[11] "Russian Federation—Strategic Weapon Systems," *Jane's Sentinel Security Assessment: Russia and the CIS*, page last updated April 16, 2020.

[12] Geoff Brumfiel, "Russia Seen Moving New Missiles to Eastern Europe," National Public Radio, December 8, 2016.

[13] As a Chinese analogue to Russia's capabilities here, Gormley et al. (2014) also posit the cost-effectiveness of a large-scale missile quiver as a complement to sustaining an active-duty combat force.

Building Tensions in the Middle East

Over the past decade, the Middle East has also seen increasing regional tension through Iran's buildup of precision missile systems. Mirroring trends in China, North Korea, and Russia, Iran has invested in expanding its missile quiver, building an inventory that rivals that of other Middle Eastern nations. The intelligence community has assessed that elements of this inventory could strike targets as far away as Europe.[14] Given that Iran has decreased its defense spending significantly since the 1980s, the buildup of its precision missile capabilities lends further credence to the argument that missile systems are increasingly viewed as worthwhile investments, with a favorable balance of cost-effectiveness and capability.

Iran has also dramatically increased the rate at which it launches missiles, both to test platforms under development and as a demonstration of capability on the world stage. Relative to the number of launches in the 1990s and early 2000s, Iranian missile launches for both testing and offensive purposes escalated significantly under the Ahmadinejad (2005–2013) and Rouhani (2013–present) regimes.[15] For example, on June 19, 2017, Iran announced that it had launched ballistic missile strikes at the Islamic State in Syria after militants targeted Tehran earlier that month.[16] Just weeks later, in July, Iran successfully launched a Simorgh missile to carry a satellite into space, signaling a significant advance in Iranian missile capabilities.[17] In January 2020, Iran exacerbated regional tensions by launching a missile salvo against U.S. forces and infrastructure at Ain al-Assad Air Base in Iraq, and in January 2021, after a day of drills involving shorter-range weapons and drones, it fired missiles against hypothetical targets almost 1,200 miles away

---

[14] "Iran—Strategic Weapon Systems," *Jane's Sentinel Security Assessment: The Gulf States*, page last updated November 1, 2020.

[15] Center for Strategic and International Studies, "Iranian Missile Launches: 1988–Present," *Missile Threat*, last updated February 10, 2020a.

[16] Artemis Moshtaghian, "Iran Launches Missiles into Eastern Syria, Targets ISIS," CNN, June 19, 2017.

[17] Thomas Erdbrink, "Iran Reports Successful Launch of Missile as U.S. Considers New Sanctions," *New York Times*, July 27, 2017.

in the Indian Ocean, which, some media outlets reported, came down 100 miles from a U.S. carrier strike group.[18] Each of these instances suggests not only Iran's interest in broadcasting its growing missile capabilities but also its willingness to employ them operationally.

Is Everything Old New Again?

While the threats, scale, and speed of a modern conflict are driving new thought in the defense community, the challenges would not be completely novel in the history of U.S. military operations. Consider, for example, U.S. airfields in the Pacific theater in World War II, where U.S. air assets and support infrastructure came under direct attack, most notably during the Japanese strikes on Hickam Field during the Pearl Harbor raid in 1941. Learning from these lessons, during the Cold War, the U.S. postured its forces in Europe to prepare for direct strikes on their operating locations. And in an effort to promote the rapid deployment of assets, the United States established and maintained a network of warehouses to store materiel in Europe, instead of housing it in centrally managed locations thousands of miles away in the continental United States.

Highlighting perceptions of an existential threat, U.S. forces emulated a large-scale attack against a NATO air base in Europe. The 1985 Salty Demo exercise simulated a Soviet bombing attack on Spangdahlem Air Base in Germany. The exercise sought to test the ability of U.S. forces to defend the base against a direct attack, to survive and recover from the attack, and to quickly restore operational capability in the wake of a bombing assault. Although most of the damage at the base was a simulacrum, the exercise incorporated some real-world elements, such as the use of actual explosives against Spangdahlem's alternate runway.[19]

---

[18] "Iran Fires Long-Range Missiles into Indian Ocean in Military Drill—Media," Reuters, January 16, 2021.

[19] For more, see John T. Correll, "Fighting Under Attack," *Air Force Magazine*, October 1, 1988.

Of course, a significant amount of time has passed since World War II and the Cold War, and, in those intervening years, the existential nature of the threat picture of those eras has faded. A key contributor has been the rarity of direct attacks on U.S. operating locations. Consequently, the lessons learned from prior decades may have been forgotten. To reinvigorate planning for the future, DoD leadership widely agrees that the defense community should actively engage in analyzing potential conflict scenarios to identify gaps and renew understanding of how to operate within a wider range of threat environments. DoD has offered formal guidance to pave the way for that planning.

The 2018 National Defense Strategy

The National Defense Strategy (NDS), published by the Office of the Secretary of Defense roughly every four years, outlines the direction that DoD will take to prepare for the global security environment in which U.S. forces will operate. The NDS itself is informed by the executive branch's national security plans and concerns, which are captured in a separate document known as the National Security Strategy.[20] As such, the NDS helps inform investments that DoD should make to modernize the force, how DoD might need to adapt its global force posture, and what changes may be warranted in amending military strategy to remain current with the evolving global security environment.

In recognition of rapidly changing threats around the globe, DoD formally acknowledged these shifts in the security environment in its latest NDS, published in 2018.[21] The strategy's focus is on preparing

---

[20] Key pillars in the latest National Security Strategy that have influenced the NDS are protecting the U.S. homeland and preserving peace through strength by renewing U.S. military capabilities. See Executive Office of the President, *National Security Strategy of the United States of America*, Washington, D.C.: White House, December 2017.

[21] U.S. Department of Defense, *Summary of the 2018 National Defense Strategy of the United States of America: Sharpening the American Military's Competitive Edge*, Washington, D.C., 2018.

for conflicts with a peer or near-peer adversary—one with comparable military capabilities to the United States. This evolution signifies a return to long-term strategic competition with such potential adversaries as China and Russia, which are seeking to erode U.S. influence and alliances and to establish their own regional dominance. Other nations, such as North Korea and Iran, are specifically highlighted in the 2018 NDS as highly capable potential adversaries, and conflict with them could stem from their efforts to destabilize the international order.

The Threat of Weapons of Mass Destruction

Although a peer or near-peer adversary could opt to use missile platforms to deliver a conventional explosive attack, the NDS identifies four other key payloads that U.S. forces could anticipate. In one such scenario, missiles could carry a chemical or biological agent. In addition to treating chemical and biological casualties with appropriate medical countermeasures, extreme precautions must be taken to ensure that any resulting contamination or contagion does not spread. Alternatively, an adversary employs a nuclear or radiological payload to yield both trauma casualties and contamination. In the case of a nuclear strike, the areal extent of the blast could yield significantly more casualties than the conventional attacks discussed thus far. An adversary's choice to employ any element from this quartet of chemical, biological, radiological, or nuclear (CBRN) options would likely be seen by U.S. leadership and by the international community as the employment of a weapon of mass destruction. The use of such a weapon could dramatically escalate the gravity, intensity, and consequences of the conflict, driving a requirement for medical resources larger than what would be expected in the wake of a conventional attack.

Such an attack—alone or in combination with a conventional missile strike—would pose complications for response efforts: A medical facility receiving CBRN casualties should be prepared to decontaminate patients before they are admitted for treatment to protect the facility's personnel and other casualties undergoing treatment. Similarly, if a biological agent is suspected, there should be a mechanism for isolating the infected to ensure its spread is restricted. With these additional requirements, the rate at which a medical facility can treat any type of patient can be expected to decline while the need for facility space, caregiver time, and medical supplies increases.

This report does not explicitly address the implications for the MHS should CBRN attacks occur on a future battlefield. One key reason is that the intelligence assessments for such attacks are rarely discussed in the open-source literature. However, the analysis exploring the implications of a conventional attack can offer a lower bound in preparing medical support for future combat operations involving CBRN attacks, with the understanding that such an attack would only escalate the need for mitigation efforts. Nonetheless, with access to the appropriate intelligence assessments, the analytic framework could be used to evaluate the medical requirements for CBRN response, available decontamination and isolation capabilities across the MHS, and the types of scenarios the MHS should prepare.

Pillars of the NDS to Prepare for Future Conflict

The NDS outlines several key endeavors that DoD must pursue to ensure that international order is maintained and that the safety, security, and economic vigor of the United States endures. It specifically calls out as core objectives the need to defend the U.S. homeland from adversary attacks and the need to defend allies against military aggression. Although, like its predecessor strategies, it highlights counterterrorism operations as relevant in the current security environment, these activities are decidedly subordinate to deterring and countering peer and near-peer threats.

The NDS outlines three lines of effort to achieve these objectives:

- *Build a more lethal force.* The military capabilities of potential adversaries rapidly increased, and the NDS emphasizes the need for the United States to modernize its military capabilities, improve its military's resilience to attack, and develop more-agile logistics and combat support capabilities that can ensure the sustained lethality of forward-deployed forces in a combat environment.
- *Strengthen alliances.* An enhanced and resilient web of allies and partners is both an important aid in deterring aggression and a

key pillar of a common defense. Thus, the United States should improve U.S. forces' interoperability with those of partner nations by investing in partner military capabilities and regularly conducting military exercises with them.

- *Reform DoD's business practices to enhance performance and affordability.* The NDS notes that DoD should operate with greater agility and cost-effectiveness. For example, it may be able to reduce its overhead costs by consolidating or restructuring duplicative business functions. In the context of acquisition, DoD's focus in recent decades has been on developing exquisite weapon systems, such as stealth fighter aircraft and high-end missile defense capabilities. This focus has led to extended development timelines and slow fielding of final systems. By amending business processes to more readily accommodate modularity and adaptability in future weapon systems, the United States will be better positioned to rapidly adapt and react to evolving adversary threats.

The 2018 NDS signifies a meaningful departure from U.S. strategies of recent decades. Consequently, defense planning and investment need to be reconsidered in response to the quickly changing global threat environment.

The Operational Implications of Adversary Missile Threats

Recognizing the change in the security environment, DoD began a broad push to better understand how to operate and succeed in future conflicts, especially those involving the use of missile systems. For example, by employing long-range ballistic and cruise missiles, an adversary could damage air bases across a theater of conflict. An adversary with these weapons could directly target key locations on runways to disrupt aircraft takeoffs and landings. Additionally, missile strikes could be directed at the parked aircraft themselves, further disrupting U.S. forces' ability to generate sorties.

These same weapon systems could be directed at other support assets to degrade combat strength. In targeting bridges and port infrastructure, such as piers, an adversary could significantly degrade U.S. freedom of movement into and within a theater of operations. If an adversary targeted fuel tank farms supporting land or maritime forces, it could restrict access to the energy resources that U.S. combat and support vehicles require. In sum, an adversary with advanced precision missile capabilities has an array of options to meaningfully degrade and disrupt U.S. combat operations.

In general, conventional missile capabilities can be thought of as an adversary's force multipliers in two key ways. Through missile strikes, an adversary could limit U.S. forces' ability to enter a combat theater (*anti-access*) and, for U.S. forces that have already deployed, limit freedom of movement to execute operations (*area denial*). This potential anti-access/area denial (A2AD) threat environment represents a fundamental change in the battlespace conditions that the U.S. military has encountered in recent decades in the Middle East.

It is worth noting that true A2AD threat conditions—fully degraded access into and within a combat theater—may be difficult for an adversary to sustain over prolonged periods. Instead, windows of opportunity for U.S. movement may appear at intervals, for example, between missile salvos or after damaged infrastructure has been repaired. Consequently, the defense community has begun to favor *contested, degraded, or operationally limited* (CDO) as the term of art in describing the restrictive conditions of the future battlefield.[22]

In scenarios typically posited by DoD experts, a high-intensity conflict under CDO conditions could be relatively short, potentially on the order of weeks. However, when U.S. forces face a degraded capability to maneuver and conduct combat and support missions, the adversary would be able to move more freely to achieve its own tactical and strategic goals and cause extensive damage to infrastructure, combat assets, and personnel.

---

[22] For more on shifts in nomenclature, see Christopher P. Cavas, "CNO Bans 'A2AD' as Jargon," *Defense News*, October 3, 2016.

The Ramifications of Heightened Missile Threats to Medical Support

DoD has clearly begun thinking about how to best posture U.S. forces and operating locations against the possible challenges of CDO, as well as necessary investments in mitigation strategies and technologies to ensure that U.S. forces can withstand and recover from attacks. In terms of withstanding an attack, defense planners seek to limit the ability of adversary missiles to engage U.S. forces. Similarly, in thinking how to recover from an attack, a planner would posit that at least some elements of an adversary's missile quiver could damage U.S. targets and consider mitigation efforts to allow U.S. forces to rapidly repair and recover from the damage.

Such mitigations could be drawn from a broad portfolio of defensive options. Some elements of this portfolio are termed *active* options, so called for their role in actively limiting an adversary's offensive capability. Examples include missile defense systems, such as Patriot missile batteries. Other contributions are considered *passive* defenses and can blunt the damaging effects of adversary missiles that successfully pass through active defense barriers. Passive options include hardened shelters to protect key assets from blasts and shrapnel; bladders and flexible hosing to disperse fuel supplies away from singular targets, such as large above-ground tanks; and concealment, camouflage, and deception technologies to confound the adversary's targeting process.[23]

However, it is important to think more broadly than just how to protect infrastructure and logistics capabilities as they come under attack. Given the explosive power of ballistic and cruise missiles, it is equally important to prepare for casualties among U.S. personnel. After all, injuries can further contribute to degraded combat capability. Consider that a cruise missile that strikes an aircraft maintenance

---

[23] For more on composing a portfolio of active and passive defense options to support force resiliency, see Brent Thomas, Mahyar A. Amouzegar, Rachel Costello, Robert A. Guffey, Andrew Karode, Christopher Lynch, Kristin F. Lynch, Ken Munson, Chad J. R. Ohlandt, Daniel M. Romano, Ricardo Sanchez, Robert S. Tripp, and Joseph V. Vesely, *Project AIR FORCE Modeling Capabilities for Support of Combat Operations in Denied Environments*, Santa Monica, Calif., RAND Corporation, RR-427-AF, 2015.

hangar can damage spare parts, support equipment, and any aircraft parked inside, among other materiel. Personnel in a deployed environment perform an array of functions to sustain overall U.S. combat capability. That same strike could also injure or kill maintenance personnel working in the hangar, runway repair personnel, engineering personnel, and others who support base operations and facilitate sortie generation, lengthening runway repair times and inhibiting U.S. forces from conducting operations (including evacuating the wounded, if necessary). Thus, medical support is a key element to consider in the overall mitigation portfolio; planning for and investing in a deployed medical capability can be as essential as procuring advanced shelters and infrastructure repair technologies.

Conclusions and Organization of This Report

This chapter provided an overview of the evolving global security environment and U.S. strategy to address these challenges, with a focus on how such potential adversaries as China, Russia, Iran, and North Korea have been investing in long-range precision missile systems. In a future conflict, potential adversaries could employ these weapons at a scale not seen before. The 2018 NDS indicates how DoD senior leaders have shifted their thinking to ensure the resilience and, ultimately, the success of U.S. forces against peer and near-peer adversaries in CDO environments. One key element of that planning falls to the MHS, which must ensure that combat casualty care can surmount the challenges that may arise in this future battlespace.

Developing a clear vision to prepare the medical community for the future of combat can be a daunting prospect. Planning for combat medical support sits at a difficult nexus. It involves integrating a diverse set of stakeholder equities, drawing on military intelligence estimates to evaluate adversary threats, interacting with medical providers to establish a list of required clinical capabilities, and drawing insights from medical logisticians to gain a larger-scale perspective on where medical practitioners will require sustainment support.

Assimilating a common sight picture across these three suites of equities will be challenging. For example, an intelligence product might describe an adversary's missile capabilities at a level of technical detail that puts it beyond the grasp of stakeholders outside this community. Clinicians tend to speak in a language of care requirements based on individual patient needs, but scaling up those requirements into plans to support large-scale trauma management might necessitate calculations by statisticians and operations research specialists. Medical logisticians benefit from a high-level synthesis of these two pictures to project storage and transport requirements to satisfy the resulting demand signals for medical support. However, logisticians might have a limited view into the handling requirements for specialty medical materiel or the risks of distributing those assets in a combat environment. They need that picture as an amalgam of the views of intelligence experts and medical clinicians. Hence, a cross-cutting assessment is needed—one that integrates multiple, diverse perspectives—to inform military planning.[24]

To explore opportunities to refine the MHS's alignment with the 2018 NDS, the remainder of this report is oriented around the series of research questions presented earlier in this chapter. Chapter One addressed how DoD's view of the global threat picture has evolved over the past decade.

In Chapter Two, the discussion continues with an overview of how the U.S. military provides care to its wounded on the battlefield and how the scale and challenges of CDO might stress the provision of care in those environments.

Chapter Three outlines a range of opportunities to adapt current medical care protocols during mass casualty events in ways that

---

[24] This is strongly reminiscent of the ancient story of the three blind men encountering an elephant for the first time. As they examine the parts of the elephant—its trunk, tail, legs—they offer very different accounts of their experiences. Moreover, they encounter great difficulty reconciling their three views. It appears that this an enduring parable of the human experience for a very good reason, given this story has been told for at least 2,500 years. See John D. Ireland, trans., *The Udana and the Itivuttaka: Two Classics from the Pali Canon*, Kandy, Sri Lanka: Buddhist Publication Society, 2007.

improve outcomes for injured warfighters, as well as where further analysis may be needed.

Chapter Four demonstrates how a renewed investigation of the costs and benefits of prepositioned medical materiel can help expedite access to key supplies and expeditionary facilities in times of need.

Chapter Five explores how the future battlefield could drive a need for enhanced resilience in medical logistics and sustainment. The discussion here presents options for staffing, partnerships, and ensuring reliable situational awareness (SA) of medical assets across the MHS network.

Through Chapter Five, the report focuses on the challenges of medical support overseas. Chapter Six instead explores the corresponding range of challenges that U.S. forces could encounter if a future fight yielded a need for large-scale casualty treatment close to and within the U.S. homeland.

Chapter Seven expands the analytic aperture to assess stressors across the medical enterprise. Specifically, it takes a closer look at the potential ramifications of large-scale casualty treatment on the industrial base for medical supplies.

Chapter Eight concludes this report with a summary of the overall insights and themes and discusses how the ramifications of the 2018 NDS might inform how the MHS prepares for a future fight.

Two appendixes provide background on the fundamental principles of triage and on the analytic models that were used to generate the findings presented in this report, respectively.

CHAPTER TWO

Challenges to Combat Casualty Care in Future Combat Operations

The previous chapter focused primarily on how threats on the battlefield are evolving. Potential adversaries, such as China, Russia, Iran, and North Korea, have made significant investments in missile technologies. The possibility that these weapons could be employed in a future conflict—particularly large-scale precision strikes from a great distance—has prompted a paradigm shift for U.S. planners and strategists. This chapter turns to the question of how those evolving threats will drive the composition of future casualty streams and how the MHS prepares to receive and treat combat casualties. To establish a baseline, the discussion begins with an overview of how combat casualties are treated today.

How the MHS Provides Care in the Conflict Environment

The standard model for the provision of medical care in expeditionary combat settings is based largely on a framework developed during U.S. deployments in the Middle East over the past two decades. The predicate of care in the deployed environment is the ability to quickly stabilize a patient's condition. Should the patient's wounds prove too severe for a return to duty after initial treatment, the patient will be evacuated to the closest MTF that offers a higher degree of treatment capability.[1]

---

[1] This represented a significant change in mindset away from one of hospital bed capacity, frequently encountered during the Cold War era. For more, see Don Snyder, Edward W. Chan, James J. Burks, Mahyar A. Amouzegar, and Adam C. Resnick, *How Should Air Force*

This sequence of stabilization, evacuation, and higher-order medical treatment can repeat, with the patient potentially evacuated from a combat theater to an MTF in the continental United States (CONUS), such as Walter Reed National Medical Center in Bethesda, Maryland. When possible, a patient will remain in theater and receive treatment until a return to duty is possible. However, if a patient's medical condition is sufficiently debilitating to *permanently* prohibit a return to duty, that patient might require a medical discharge from the service. In the case of the gravest injuries, that patient could die. This process of patient treatment and flow is presented in Figure 2.1.

In this paradigm of care, at the POI, injured personnel initially receive basic first aid. This level of care can be provided by either a fellow soldier or the injured patient (self-help first aid). During training, service members learn such fundamental medical skills as bandaging a wound and applying a tourniquet. Should medical interventions at the POI prove inadequate for the patient to return to duty, the patient will receive successively higher levels of medical care. These levels of medical capability are also referred to as *roles* or *echelons* of care.

It is important to highlight another core medical capability, known as *en route care*, in which patients are tended by a medical team in transit between medical facilities. En route care is not generally con-

Figure 2.1
Framework for Providing Care in Expeditionary Environments

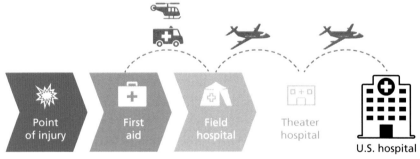

Expeditionary Medical Capabilities Be Expressed? Santa Monica, Calif.: RAND Corporation, MG-785-AF, 2009.

sidered a separate echelon of treatment, but the capabilities of medical teams that travel with patients do scale relative to the severity of a patient's condition. Consequently, en route care is considered an integral component of the medical support a patient may receive during a course of treatment.

In the network of MTFs where a patient receives treatment, medical facilities are designated according to one of four formal roles of care. This role assignment is based on the medical support available at the MTF:[2]

- *Role 1* is generally the first level of medical care a combat casualty will receive. These unit-level MTFs tend to be small and lightly staffed, providing personnel with prevention services and treating disease and non-battle injuries. For those who have been wounded in combat, a Role 1 facility can offer basic resuscitation and stabilization of trauma injuries prior to the patient's evacuation to a higher echelon of care.
- *Role 2* care offers enhanced expeditionary medical capabilities and throughput for emergency medical services and trauma care. For example, Role 2 facilities might offer basic x-ray services and stock an array of blood and blood products for transfusion. A Role 2 MTF can be equipped with varying degrees of surgical capability and holding capacity for intensive care patients.
- *Role 3* further builds out the medical services offered at Role 2 facilities, providing additional types of specialty and ancillary care, such as orthopedic surgery and basic physical therapy. To support combat casualties, Role 3 facilities also offer an expanded suite of surgical services and additional capacity to hold intensive care patients.
- *Role 4* care features the most expansive suite of medical capabilities. In addition to expanded trauma, surgical, and intensive care support, Role 4 facilities offer definitive care and rehabilitation

---

[2] For a more detailed exploration of roles of care, refer to Joint Publication 4-02, *Joint Health Services*, Washington, D.C.: U.S. Joint Chiefs of Staff, incorporating change 1, September 28, 2018.

services. Consequently, Role 4 is associated with larger MTFs in CONUS, such as Walter Reed, and some advanced overseas facilities, such as Landstuhl Regional Medical Center in Germany.

From this foundation in how the MHS delivers care to those wounded in combat, we next turn our attention to the assessment of the types of injuries the MTF network might receive.

Estimating Injury Types in a Future Fight

To frame the risk to personnel in a future combat environment, it is important to first consider the injury patterns stemming from adversary weapon systems. As noted in Chapter One, a principal pathway for injury would be a ballistic or cruise missile explosion. Although U.S. forces have not encountered blast environments at scale involving these weapons, there are analogues from recent history that can help estimate the injury patterns and frequencies U.S. forces could encounter on the future battlefield.

A contemporary analogue is the injury signature of smaller conventional explosives. For example, during contingency support during Operation Iraqi Freedom and Operation Enduring Freedom in Afghanistan, U.S. forces were injured in blast events involving mortars, rocket-propelled grenades, and improvised explosive devices. A missile would likely carry an explosive payload far larger than the weapons commonly employed in Iraq and Afghanistan, but weaponeering analysis suggests that the distribution of injury types will not differ significantly. The most distinctive is that a missile's larger net explosive weight would result in a greater radius of effect. Consequently, each blast can cause a significantly larger number of casualties.[3]

---

[3] Several assessments have examined conditions under which injury distributions remain reasonably constant but casualty numbers occur at greater scale. See, for example, Trevor N. Dupuy, *The Evolution of Weapons and Warfare*, Fairfax, Va.: Hero Books, 1984, and Richard A. Gabriel and Karen S. Metz, *A History of Military Medicine*, 2 vols., New York: Greenwood Press, 1992.

To support planning for medical needs during future combat operations, the Naval Health Research Center has collated relevant historical injury profiles in a database known as the Patient Condition Occurrence Frequency (PCOF) tool. The center's casualty modeling software, the Medical Planners' Toolkit (MPTk), houses a range of PCOF data, including those from historical combat and disaster relief operations.[4] The injuries described in recent combat injury PCOF data include those sustained during Operation Iraqi Freedom and Operation Enduring Freedom. In these cases, personnel who were farthest from the blast frequently had moderate injuries (as measured on the Abbreviated Injury Scale). In comparison, injuries received closer to the POI were more likely to be life-threatening. These wounds ranged from modest limb fractures to critical injuries, such as multiple amputations and open skull fractures.

It is important to note that the Abbreviated Injury Scale categories do not occur in equal measure in the historical records. This becomes more intuitive when approaching the problem from a geometric perspective. Consider the relative areas of blast effects, as depicted in Figure 2.2. The area of effect for generating moderate injuries (with a radius far from the point of detonation) is significantly greater than the area where more critical injuries are expected (with a radius close to the point of detonation). As the net explosive payload of a weapon increases, the three radii of effect in the figure simply extend farther away from the center of the detonation.

These relative effects are borne out in the historical data, as shown in Figure 2.3. From the PCOF data on conventional blast munitions, roughly 83 percent of personnel have historically received moderate, non–life-threatening injuries, while 17 percent of patients fall into the serious, severe, and critical categories. Many patients with these graver injuries will likely require significant surgical intervention to save their

---

Weaponeering techniques offer methods for extrapolating blast effects as net explosive weights increase. See Craig Payne, *Principles of Naval Weapons Systems*, 2nd ed., Annapolis, Md.: Naval Institute Press, 2010.

[4] MPTk's range of capabilities is documented in Naval Health Research Center, "Medical Planners' Toolkit (MPTk): Medical Mission Support," San Diego, Calif., 2013b.

Figure 2.2
Notional Depiction of Injury Severity and Distance from a Blast Event

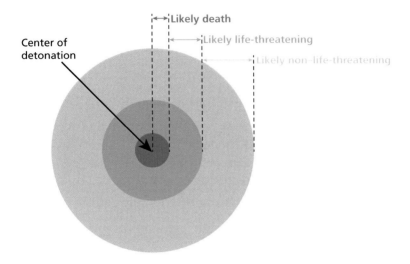

Figure 2.3
Historical Injury Distribution Due to Conventional Explosives

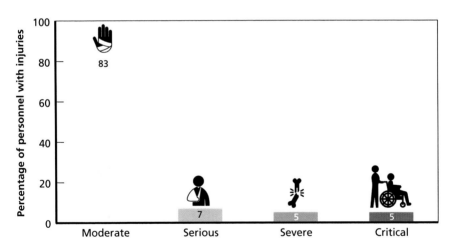

SOURCE: Naval Health Research Center data on blast events during Operation
Enduring Freedom–Afghanistan and Operation Iraqi Freedom, 2006–2014.

lives. At first glance, the prospect of more than 80 percent of patients presenting with recoverable injuries seems promising for care in the deployed environment. However, the remainder of patients who are more gravely injured can stress—if not overwhelm—available medical care capacity in the field, especially when the overall size of the casualty population is large.

Using this framework for predicting the relative severities and types of injuries from a large-scale blast event, the next section examines how many personnel are at risk of being injured in a missile strike.

Linking the Missile Targeting Problem to the Number of Injured

As one might imagine, the adversary's decisionmaking process is central to estimating how many personnel may be injured in a strike. Casualty rates depend on the adversary's choice of targets. Consider, for example, that an adversary opts to attack an airfield supporting U.S. operations. At a typical airfield, there are very few personnel in runway areas and near fuel farms at any given time. In a deployed environment, munitions bunkers and missile defense systems are likely to have more personnel working at their duty stations. In comparison, aircraft parking and maintenance areas are some of the more populous areas on base.

However, understanding where personnel are located at a base is only part of the equation. It is just as important to understand what target sets an adversary considers important enough to damage and advance progress toward strategic aims. The adversary must make crucial targeting choices that further a paramount operational goal, such as the sustained suppression of U.S. sortie generation at the airfield. The adversary targeting problem involves a complex calculus of assessing not only what assets are involved in the support of air power but also the inherent reparability or recovery of those assets after they are attacked.

Further complicating these calculations, an adversary targeteer must pay careful attention to the size of the missile inventory. While apportioning missiles to targets, the targeteer must account for the like-lihood of a successful strike, which could be affected by the accuracy of the weapon systems and the availability and effectiveness of local missile defense systems. These factors must be weighed against the number of missiles required to successfully deny access to the targeted asset. For example, in targeting runways, it is essential to consider both the number and location of points on the runway that must be success-fully damaged to prevent aircraft takeoffs and landings. Furthermore, as noted earlier, the targeteer would also account for available runway repair capability at the airfield, which can inform the required fre-quency of missile strikes to ensure that the runway remains unavailable for flight operations.

Figure 2.4 illustrates one of many possible targeting choices. In this notional targeting plan, the adversary has chosen to levy a signifi-cant strike against a base's aircraft parking area in an effort to damage as many aircraft on the ground as possible. The secondary goal involves

Figure 2.4
Notional Adversary Targeting Plan Against an Air Operating Location

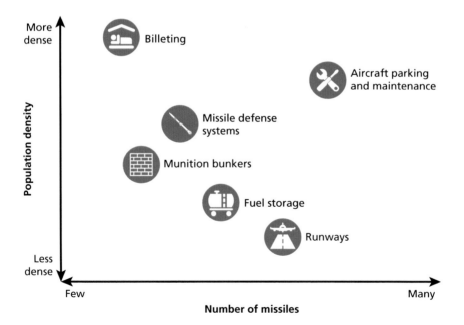

damaging runway surfaces and destroying fuel reserves to limit sorties by any surviving aircraft. Other base targets, such as munitions stores, missile defenses, and billeting, played a much smaller role in this notional targeting plan, as they were seen as tertiary in their support for airpower generation. Note that this is just one possible targeting plan against a single notional airfield. The adversary must complete similar plans for every other operating location in the theater, giving rise to potentially complex resource management decisions, as discussed earlier.

Figure 2.4 also highlights an important feature of targeting plans—namely, relative population density. This is a key dimension for U.S. military planners as they estimate the potential requirements for medical care prior to deploying to a combat theater. Ultimately, it may be impossible to precisely calculate how much medical support should be available in a given location, because there is a great deal of uncertainty about what an adversary will strike, at what time, and with how many munitions. Consequently, it is important to embrace and incorporate uncertainty into the estimation process. For example, uncertainty might be accounted for by evaluating a range of targeting plans to gain an understanding of the potential range of an adversary's weapon systems. In tandem, this calculation will also inform estimates of casualty numbers. This robust decisionmaking process can help map out the complex tradespace of operational effects, providing senior leadership with a more complete and nuanced awareness of potential outcomes.[5]

After estimating the size and extent of possible casualty streams in the combat environment, a medical planner is still left with a few key questions. Namely, how might the network of expeditionary MTFs process patient loads at a scale and scope likely to be encountered in

---

[5] For more on the importance of explicitly incorporating uncertainty in policy analysis, see Paul K. Davis and Steven W. Popper, "Confronting Model Uncertainty in Policy Analysis for Complex Systems: What Policymakers Should Demand," *Journal on Policy and Complex Systems*, Vol. 5, No. 2, Fall 2019.

For more on a modeling approach for incorporating uncertain targeting strategies into the selection of a resiliency portfolio, see Thomas et al., 2015.

future combat? The next section explores patient outcomes in this environment.

Core Challenges to Medical Support in a Future Fight

It should be clear from the discussion thus far that the U.S. military has very agile, modular, and scalable medical support. Historically, during Operation Iraqi Freedom and Operation Enduring Freedom, the available network of Role 1, 2, and 3 capabilities enabled an efficient process for stabilizing and treating patients, and any needed subsequent evacuation of patients to a higher echelon of care could happen quickly and efficiently. Overall, during these two operations, the availability of expeditionary medical care ensured that more than 90 percent of those wounded survived.[6] Excellent historical patient outcomes stemmed in large part from rapid access to medical personnel and materiel, an assumption often stated in military planning documents.[7] Based on the historical patient loads in these conflicts, with sufficient access to evacuation assets and advances in the rapid stabilization of trauma patients, it may be possible to further shrink the footprint of in-theater MTFs on the ground and accelerate the evacuation of patients who require more care.

There are, however, key predicates that may belie their relevance to medical support in the face of evolving threats. For example, in the aftermath of a large-scale missile attack, the number of patients requiring trauma care could exceed the available capacity of expeditionary MTFs. In concert, it may be difficult to assign patients to space on board a limited number aeromedical evacuation platforms. Further-

---

[6] This metric is also known as the case fatality rate. For more on the range of commonly used combat casualty care statistics, see John B. Holcomb, Lynn G. Stansbury, Howard R. Champion, Charles Wade, and Ronald F. Bellamy, "Understanding Combat Casualty Care Statistics," *Journal of Trauma*, Vol. 60, No. 2, February 2006.

[7] For example, this is a predicate in current Air Force planning. See Air Force Tactics, Techniques, and Procedures 3-42.71, *Expeditionary Medical Support (EMEDS) and Air Force Theater Hospital (AFTH)*, Washington, D.C.: U.S. Department of the Air Force, August 27, 2014.

more, the locations of undamaged airfields might not coincide with where the patients are located. Thus, the historical quality of and access to U.S. expeditionary medical support over the past several decades reflects the security conditions of the time—a threat that yielded a relatively small patient load and a security environment that offered the United States freedom of movement, especially by air.[8] These are the very assumptions that must be challenged when planning for CDO environments.

The set of difficulties that the MHS could face during large-scale combat operations will likely come down to a connected web of three factors: capacity, capability, and throughput. In terms of capacity, expeditionary MTFs would likely see surges of trauma patients, and they might need to hold more patients than expected, both during and after treatment. To reduce strain, MTFs could increase the throughput of patients. Consequently, the MHS will need to consider mechanisms that can accelerate the rate at which medical personnel at expeditionary MTFs can stabilize and treat casualties, perform lifesaving procedures, and expedite patient evacuation to higher echelons of care, as needed. Finally, given that future large-scale combat operations could yield a larger number of severe trauma patients, MTF capacity and capabilities might need to be expanded. For example, augmenting the staff and resources needed to perform surgeries at smaller MTFs might lead to meaningful improvements in patient outcomes.

Over the past few years, a growing number of defense analysts, medical professionals, and military planners have voiced concerns about these possible challenges in supporting future combat operations. These concerns are wide-ranging but touch on the core hallmarks of capacity, throughput, and capability, as well as the need for the MHS to invest in enhancing these pillars of expeditionary military support. The following are some perspectives from the published literature:

---

[8]   For a broader historical view of evolving requirements for casualty care spanning two centuries of U.S. combat support, see Bernard D. Rostker, *Providing for the Casualties of War: The American Experience Through World War II*, Santa Monica, Calif.: RAND Corporation, MG-1164-OSD, 2013.

Over the course of a protracted series of missile strikes, the resulting trauma casualties would yield a long-term, large-scale demand signal for blood. Furthermore, these same strikes would limit the timely movement of blood into the theater from donation centers and warehouses in the continental United States. As the conflict wears on, blood in local storage at medical treatment facilities across the theater could be depleted, leading to challenges in providing blood in sufficient quantity to combat casualties.[9]

By basing planning on lessons from recent small-scale combat operations, we are at risk of shaping the medical force out to 2028 in ways that will make [large-scale combat operations] medically unsupportable.[10]

Provision of medical support could be a worthy priority for NATO planners when considering deterrence of and defense against near-peer or peer adversaries. . . . Dealing with advanced A2AD threats and ensuring NATO's ability to deter, defend, and conduct operations will therefore require both political and military leaders to invest in medical support.[11]

One of the great success stories in today's golden hour care is the reintroduction and revamping of the tourniquet, after decades of disuse because of antiquated designs and a poor understanding of how it was to be optimally used. . . . The history of the tourniquet is a reminder that, just as military strategy and tactics need to change as new wars are fought against new adversaries, so too do technologies, procedures, and beliefs surrounding medical care.[12]

---

[9] Brent Thomas, Katherine Anania, Anthony DeCicco, and John A. Hamm, *Toward Resiliency in the Joint Blood Supply Chain*, Santa Monica, Calif.: RAND Corporation, RR-2482-DARPA, 2018, p. xi.

[10] F. Cameron Jackson, "Don't Get Wounded: Military Health System Consolidation and the Risk to Readiness," *Military Review*, September–October 2019, p. 142.

[11] Marta Kepe, "Lives on the Line: The A2AD Challenge to Combat Casualty Care," Modern War Institute at West Point, July 30, 2018.

[12] Tanisha M. Fazal, Todd Rasmussen, Paul Nelson, and P. K. Carlton, "How Long Can the U.S. Military's Golden Hour Last?" *War on The Rocks*, October 8, 2018. Recall that *golden*

Ultimately, [medical support to combat operations in denied environments] is not a medical problem. It is a line issue directly related to combat capability and the use of [service], Joint, and Coalition medical capabilities to ensure that the human element within the Military instrument of power remains quantitatively and qualitatively viable for combat operations.[13]

Conclusions

The chapter began with a discussion of how the MHS delivers care in the deployed environment. By quickly stabilizing, treating, and evacuating wounded service members, the MHS has seen tremendous success in reducing fatalities and improving outcomes after injuries. However, the current posture of medical support has evolved in a way that is optimized for past operations, with light patient loads and an assumption that U.S. forces will have air superiority to safely evacuate patients to higher echelons of care, as needed. The 2018 NDS emphasizes a need to prepare for large-scale combat operations, and these assumptions may no longer consistently apply.

Adversary weapon systems, such as ballistic and cruise missiles, could yield large numbers of blast casualties. In tandem, by targeting the infrastructure that supports military mobility, an adversary can readily degrade the U.S. forces' freedom of movement. Under such future combat conditions, these factors could tax or overwhelm the capacity, capability, and throughput of deployed military medical care. The next chapter begins to explore potential opportunities for the MHS to alleviate these types of constraints in caring for future combat casualties.

---

hour refers to when a seriously injured trauma patient has a higher likelihood of survival with quick medical intervention, nominally within one hour. For more, see R. A. Cowley, "A Total Emergency Medical System for the State of Maryland," *Maryland State Medical Journal*, Vol. 24, No. 7, July 1975.

[13] Patrick B. Parsons, *Medical Support for Combat Operations in a Denied Environment (MS-CODE): Considerations for Immediate and Future Operations and Research Across the Strategic, Operational, and Tactical Domains*, Maxwell Air Force Base, Ala.: Air War College, April 6, 2017, p. 31.

CHAPTER THREE

Enhancing Care on the Future Battlefield

The MHS delivers quality medical care to service members wounded in combat, with special attention to rapidly stabilizing combat casualties and, as needed, swiftly evacuating the injured to an echelon of care appropriate for their wounds. However, the security environment outlined in the 2018 NDS suggests that, in a future fight with a peer or near-peer adversary, the military's expeditionary care network could be overwhelmed by large numbers of casualties. In such a conflict, not only could the military see a significantly degraded ability to treat large numbers of combat wounded, but it could also encounter significant declines in operational capabilities while the wounded are awaiting treatment or recovering.

This chapter turns to a logical follow-on question: How might expeditionary medical care providers be better prepared to handle future casualties at large scale? Improvements in three key domains could help expedite and improve care under these conditions: the capability, capacity, and throughput of the expeditionary care network. Across this triad, the MHS could pursue an array of mitigations, starting with care at the POI.

Enhancing Training for First Responders

As discussed in Chapter Two, at the POI, the first line of treatment could be the patient or a nearby service member. All military forces receive training in basic first aid. For example, through the Air Force's tactical combat casualty care curriculum, airmen learn such fundamentals as bandaging, tourniquet use, and heat stroke mitigation. Commenting on the value of POI care during combat operations in Afghanistan, historian of military medicine Emily Mayhew remarked, "Bring a medic, bring a hospital, but above all bring a soldier's own understanding of what he needs to do to his own point of wounding."[1]

This type of training is necessary because there are limited numbers of medically trained first responders, such as Navy hospital corpsmen and Air Force independent-duty medical technicians. Given the types and severity of injuries likely to be seen in future conflict environments, basic first aid skills may be insufficient to stabilize or treat patients at the POI.

As an alternative, the MHS might elect to augment this basic medical training with a broader suite of first response capabilities for selected service members. While it may prove too expensive to train all service members to a more capable standard than basic first aid, the services could target training opportunities toward those in occupations at higher risk of combat injury in a future large-scale conflict, including not only front-line combat personnel but also key support staff, such as combat vehicle maintainers and civil engineers.

One such standard is the U.S. Army's combat lifesaver training protocol. Trainees learn critical lifesaving interventions beyond those taught in basic first aid programs, such as Air Force tactical combat casualty care. The Army's combat lifesaver curriculum features two key medical interventions that could have great utility in a POI combat casualty care scenario. First, trainees learn advanced hemorrhage control, both with and without a tourniquet. Then, they are trained to employ needle decompression to treat tension pneumothorax, a life-threatening condition caused by blast fragmentation or shrapnel lacerating the lungs.

Enhancing the skills of first responders could lead to meaningful decreases in the number of patients who succumb to their wounds at the POI and increases in the number of gravely wounded patients who survive and seek admission to nearby Role 2 field hospitals. These

---

[1]   Emily Mayhew, *A Heavy Reckoning: War, Medicine, and Survival in Afghanistan and Beyond*, London: Profile Books, 2017.

patients will require further treatment and, likely, surgical care, further taxing the limited resources at these small MTFs. Consequently, this heightened demand could drive a need for additional evacuation resources, thereby cascading strain across the deployed network of care.

Nonetheless, the MHS should consider further enhancing the medical skill sets of those most likely to offer first-line care on the battlefield. However, it will need to ensure that the training is effective and cost-effective, so that the program is sustainable. The first step is to identify the target population for an advanced first aid program, which could be front-line combat support personnel; combat service support personnel, such as logisticians and maintainers; or all military deployers. The cost of the training program can be assessed based on the target population and the cost offset relative to their current medical training platforms. The results of this assessment could inform the development of specialized technology, such as a handheld rapid-diagnosis system, among other investments to promote the effectiveness and cost-effectiveness of enhanced first aid.

Augmenting Expeditionary Medical Treatment Facilities

The previous section discussed the potential benefits to patient outcomes in enhancing first responder capabilities at the POI. But what if Role 2 MTFs that receive these patients are already at or near capacity? Additional mitigations will likely be needed to limit the necessity to queue patients who require care at expeditionary field hospitals. One such mitigation would be a mechanism to expand the capacity of field hospitals. In thinking about the possibility of capacity expansion, it is worth examining the modularity of expeditionary MTFs.

As noted in Chapter Two, each of the U.S. military services has a deployable medical capability that can support a variety of operations. Across this spectrum of medical support, each service devotes significant attention to providing care for casualties incurred during combat operations. To do so, the services have developed large deployable MTFs, such as Army combat support hospitals, Navy expeditionary medical facility, and Air Force theater hospitals. These facilities can provide a wide array of medical services to the deployed population, including public health services, force health protection, and care for injuries sustained during both combat and steady-state operations.

Over its extended operations in the Middle East, the Air Force developed a modular medical capability to enable more-rapid deployment and to increase efficiency in support of smaller operations. These MTFs, collectively known as the Expeditionary Medical Support (EMEDS) system, can be scaled up to meet anticipated patient loads and to provide the range of medical services that patients may require. For example, expanding the default four-bed EMEDS health response team, the ten-bed EMEDS+10 configuration receives augmentation for patient holding support, surgical and critical care, and additional laboratory and medical logistics support.

Given the success of the EMEDS construct over the past two decades, other services are pursuing a similar degree of modularity in their expeditionary medical capabilities, such as the Navy's drive to develop a capability-based MTF and the Army's current push to fractionate its large combat support hospital capability into smaller building blocks.[2] This modularity will give the services greater freedom to customize and tailor expeditionary medical capabilities to better meet operational requirements with a lighter, smaller footprint. The ability to structure and equip MTFs in such a fashion—collating capabilities based on anticipated need for care—can provide each of the services with a flexible and agile mechanism for highly capable medical response.

In other words, the MHS has deployable medical facilities capable of scaling to accommodate patient loads. The modular framework of some MTFs, including the Air Force EMEDS, readily allows for this in a materiel sense. From there, tentage and support equipment can be added to expand the field hospital with additional ward beds, operating rooms, or intensive care units. The expansion of medical facilities would likely also require concomitant augmentation of facility person-

---

[2]   The Army has begun to convert its 248-bed CSHs to more-modular field hospitals, where core medical capabilities could be augmented with 32-bed surgical, 24-bed medical, and 60-bed intermediate care ward detachments.

nel, with more physicians, surgeons, nurses, and technicians deploying to populate the expanded MTF.

Both materiel and personnel mitigations may be possible, but careful thought is warranted during planning. In a resource-constrained environment, procuring additional materiel can prove challenging, and the costs associated with training and retention of skilled medical personnel could prove prohibitive. Alternatively, the services may be able to partner to achieve desired augmentation goals. For example, should the Air Force note that the likely demand for care exceeds its footprint in a combat theater, the Army might be able to augment selected MTFs with soldiers from its regional supply of caregivers and medical providers or with elements of one of its unused combat support hospitals.

Analysis has shown that, with expanded field hospital capacity, patient queues at crowded MTFs can significantly decrease. With the ability to admit additional patients with non–life-threatening wounds, such an MTF can aid in accelerating return-to-duty rates. Equally significantly, with an increase in the capacity to hold patients with life-threatening injuries, a key benefit is a significant drop in the number of patients who die of their wounds. It is worth noting that there could be a resulting increase in the number of stabilized patients who require definitive care, which increases the demand signal for evacuation to a higher-echelon MTF.[3]

Introducing Concussion Protocols

So far, the mitigations discussed have focused on improving the provision of care, especially for the benefit of trauma patients in the casualty streams arriving at expeditionary MTFs. However, it is also important to consider the patient population as a whole to determine whether there are specific injury types in the record of blast victims that warrant additional attention in planning for mass casualty events.

---

[3] For an example of these effects through the lens of a simulated EMEDS, see John A. Hamm, *Improving the Air Force Medical Service's Expeditionary Medical Support System: A Simulation Approach: Analysis of Mass-Casualty Combat and Disaster Relief Scenarios*, dissertation, Santa Monica, Calif.: RAND Corporation, RGSD-A343-1, 2020.

Recall from Figure 2.3 in Chapter Two that approximately 80 percent of the blast casualty population suffers from non–life-threatening injuries. A more in-depth look at the Naval Health Research Center's blast injury PCOF (the source of the data in Figure 2.3) indicates that roughly half of these personnel had some form of concussion. Categorized broadly, these injuries are often referred to as *mild traumatic brain injury* (mTBI). A growing body of evidence indicates that many mTBI patients can recover on their own and return to duty gradually over the course of a few days.[4] Under the watchful eye of a fellow service member, patients can return to quarters until they have recovered sufficiently to return to duty. However, if their symptoms fail to ameliorate in that time, treatment at an MTF may be warranted. Consequently, patients and those watching over them in quarters need to be alert to key concussion symptoms, such as an extreme sensitivity to light or sound, and seek medical care for the patient if those symptoms persist or worsen.

According to Naval Health Research Center data, many combat casualties awaiting care at an MTF will likely have an mTBI. Given that many mTBI patients recover on their own with limited medical intervention, it may be useful to introduce a triage strategy to segregate mTBI patients from the general patient population. In such a strategy, patients would be able to return to barracks or light duty, returning to the MTF in the event that their symptoms worsen. Such a strategy would lead to meaningful reductions in the queue of patients awaiting treatment. Table 3.1 presents a notional concussion recovery proto-

---

[4]   Carrie M. Farmer, Heather Krull, Thomas W. Concannon, Molly M. Simmons, Francesca Pillemer, Teague Ruder, Andrew M. Parker, Maulik P. Purohit, Liisa Hiatt, Benjamin Saul Batorsky, and Kimberly A. Hepner, *Understanding Treatment of Mild Traumatic Brain Injury in the Military Health System*, Santa Monica, Calif.: RAND Corporation, RR-844-OSD, 2016.

In the case of the 2020 Iranian missile strike on Ain al-Asad, more than 100 U.S. service members suffered concussion injuries, with most returning to duty within a few days. The absence of other trauma injuries as a result of the strike stemmed from the availability of sufficient warning for personnel to take cover. For more, see Idrees Ali and Phil Stewart, "More Than 100 U.S. Troops Diagnosed with Brain Injuries from Iran Attack," Reuters, February 10, 2020.

Table 3.1
Notional Concussion Patient Recovery Protocol

Patient State	Outcome	Safe Activities
No symptoms after mandatory 24-hour rest and exertion test	Return to pre-injury activity	Patient may return to duty and resume all activities.
Symptomatic after 24 hours	Additional 24 hours of rest	Patient may not return to duty until the next symptom check at 48 hours.
Symptomatic after 48 hours	Progressive return to duty over the course of 5 days	Further analysis is needed to determine appropriate options.

SOURCE: Defense and Veterans Brain Injury Center, "DoD Clinical Recommendation: Progressive Return to Activity Following Acute Concussion/Mild Traumatic Brain Injury: Guidance for the Primary Care Manager in Deployed and Non-Deployed Settings," Arlington, Va.: Defense Centers of Excellence for Psychological Health and Traumatic Brain Injury, January 2014.

col which incorporates clinical recommendations and guidelines as to when mTBI patients can return to duty.[5]

A concussion triage protocol in the aftermath of a large-scale casualty event would need to build upon two fundamental interventions. The first would be to increase service members' awareness of concussion symptoms and associated recovery timelines. Doing so will help them both self-assess for mTBI and watch for symptoms in others. This suite of signs and symptoms could be added to fundamental first aid curricula as a special mTBI awareness unit. The second intervention would be to map an appropriate path for a recovering mTBI patient to return to duty, something that would require additional research. For example, reassignment to loading weapons onto combat vehicles could prove too strenuous, and a vehicle maintenance center could be too noisy. Hence, alternative duty stations may be needed for recovering patients; further assessment can inform the development of formal protocols for returning to duty in the aftermath of a concussion injury.

---

[5] More information on concussion protocols can be found in Defense and Veterans Brain Injury Center, 2014.

Adapting Treatment Prioritization During Mass Trauma Events

As discussed, the introduction of a triage strategy that can separate patients with non–life-threatening mTBI from the general casualty population holds promise for reducing congestion at field hospitals. Moreover, this strategy, coupled with a straightforward recovery protocol for concussion patients, can expedite return-to-duty. Given the potential benefits of triage in reducing patient load at MTFs and in improving mTBI patient outcomes, it might be useful to think through how triage strategies could benefit medical outcomes for patients with a higher mortality risk.

As suggested earlier, even if mTBI patients are directed away from treatment facilities, many field hospitals could still be overwhelmed by the number of patients awaiting treatment and by the required medical support needs to tend to their wounds. The key concern is that, during a large-scale casualty event, the magnitude of patient surges could exceed a facility's capacity to help all those in need of medical attention. In such a scenario, once mTBI patients have been screened out of the patient population, the remaining casualty stream might be more accurately described as stemming from a mass trauma rather than mass casualty event.[6]

A mass trauma scenario would provide a unique set of challenges at an MTF, especially at a small Role 2 facility. For example, the medical provider and caregiver staff will have little to no slack capacity in their workload. Moreover, key treatment areas at a field hospital, such as the operating theater and the intensive care ward, can expect full utilization. And a facility's critical medical supplies, especially pain medications and blood products, may need to be carefully managed.

---

[6] In a *mass casualty* scenario, a medical facility or hospital provides treatment to a spike or sustained surge of patients with any medical condition. This population could include patients with injuries, from mTBI to severe wounds, as well as with contagious conditions, such as flu or COVID-19.

In a *mass trauma* scenario, a facility or hospital admits only the most injured patients for treatment. This type of scenario can be more demanding for medical providers and facilities: The need for intervention is more urgent, the treatment timelines are longer, and the demand for supplies—especially blood, in the case of blast victims—skyrockets.

During casualty surge events, however, decisions about how to appropriately triage patients may be challenging. Given the history and success of medical support to military operations in the Middle East over the past few decades, many medical personnel have only been exposed to patient streams in which all injured personnel in need of care could be seen by a medical provider. Even during patient surges, by prioritizing admission for those with the most critical injuries, field hospital staff could frequently still triage patients in a way that allowed them to treat all patients in need of medical care.

In the aftermath of a mass trauma event, focusing limited medical staff, facilities, and supplies on a few of the most critically injured would quickly outstrip each available resource. Therein lies the crux of the decision for medical providers: With limited resources, should one prioritize care for a few of the critically injured or offer critical patients palliative services while directing the bulk of care to those with severe injuries?[7] This decision is at the heart of medical triage: Relative to the limited availability of scarce medical resources, how must one sort and prioritize patients to ensure the best possible outcomes for the overall patient population?[8] It is important to note that critically injured patients are those at highest risk of mortality, *even with treatment.* This high expectation of mortality is especially salient given the resource limitations at small field hospitals.[9]

Simulation analysis can help inform outcomes at a field hospital facing a surge demand of non-concussion blast injury victims. Figure 3.1 depicts characteristic simulation outcomes after changes in treatment prioritization during a mass trauma event at a Role 2 MTF.

---

[7] In the context of nomenclature used in the Abbreviated Injury Scale, a *critical* injury is one with high severity and a high risk of mortality, such as an open skull fracture. A *serious* injury is less severe and offers a lower risk of mortality, such as an open humerus fracture.

[8] Given the centrality of triage in the provision of care during a mass casualty event, Appendix A offers a more in-depth exploration of this core problem set.

[9] Although the discussion here focuses on the context of military support to casualties, extreme circumstances have dictated the careful rationing of trauma care in the civilian sector as well. For a journalist's account of support at an overwhelmed civilian facility during Serbia's siege of Srebrenica between 1992 and 1995, see Sheri Lee Fink, *War Hospital: A True Story of Surgery and Survival*, New York: Perseus Books, 2003.

Figure 3.1
The Role of Treatment Priority in Simulated Patient Outcomes and Blood Requirements at a Role 2 MTF During a Mass Trauma Casualty Surge

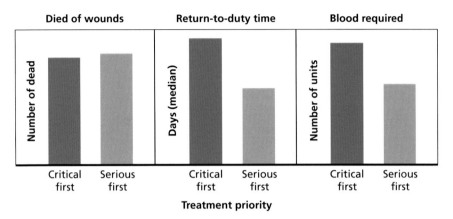

SOURCE: Analysis relied on the Naval Health Research Center's MPTk and Joint Medical Planning Tool (JMPT), which simulates patient flows through a user-designed network of care based on extant MHS capabilities.

NOTES: Specific numerical outcomes depend on the number and timing of casualty arrivals, as well as the capacity and capability of the receiving MTF. Results in the figure are representative of a Role 2 facility receiving more than 100 patients. For more specifics, including outcomes at larger MTFs, see Hamm, 2020.

If the treatment priority follows the more common expectation that the most critically injured are seen and treated first, a meaningful number of the total patient population can be expected to succumb to their wounds. This is a consequence of the frequency and gravity of injuries across the population of blast victims. Resources at the field hospital are insufficient to guarantee the survivability of the entire patient population.

Figure 3.1 also highlights how return-to-duty times can be slow among a patient population. Here, the primary focus of caregivers' time will be treating the most gravely injured patients rather than patients who are more likely to return to duty quickly after non–life-threatening wounds. Furthermore, given that the critical trauma patients have a probable need for massive transfusions, the requirement for blood products can be quite significant.

Figure 3.1 also depicts the consequence of initially providing palliative care to the most critically injured while directing remaining caregiver time toward treating the population of seriously injured patients. The figure shows that, under this triage strategy, the number of patients who would die of their wounds may increase slightly. However, under this prioritization strategy, a large fraction of caregiver time and facility resources can be allocated to treating patients with non–life-threatening wounds. This significantly reduces the median return-to-duty time for the overall patient population.

By accelerating the reconstitution of the force, patients who return to duty promptly can offer important benefits in ensuring an operating location's safety. For example, the rapid return of combat teams and vehicle maintainers to their duty stations can contribute to the recovery of operational capability. Similarly, returning missile defense personnel to duty would help restore the ability to intercept inbound missiles. This triage strategy can also reduce the demand for blood products, allowing for a reserve of critical supplies to treat casualties in the aftermath of future attacks.

Selecting an appropriate triage strategy can mean rapidly making life-or-death decisions for patients, especially when the number of people who urgently need medical attention can vastly outstrip available resources. Furthermore, adapting an appropriate triage strategy can be extremely difficult in peacetime conditions, let alone during conflict. For example, difficult treatment priority decisions were made in the wake of Hurricane Katrina, where the operating environment mimicked CDO conditions. The hurricane's disruptions included power outages, limited freedom of movement for ambulances, restricted access to an overtaxed air ambulance fleet, downed communication lines, diminishing and spoiling supplies, and even the perception of looting risk at hospitals. In such stressful circumstances, especially when triage skills have gone unpracticed, practitioners may spend valuable time trying to determine appropriate triage strategies as patient flows surge.[10] However, if triage is routinely practiced, facil-

---

[10] Fink drew similar conclusions, most notably in her book *Five Days at Memorial: Life and Death in a Storm-Ravaged Hospital*, New York: Crown Publishers, 2013.

ity staff will be better prepared to do the most good for the largest number of patients even with limited resources. Patient outcomes will then improve as a result of efficient processing, sorting, and prioritizing of medical resources to best align with the needs of the patient population.

It is important to note that most medical facilities, both civilian and military, do indeed practice triage protocols. However, the training event that frames these drills typically revolves around disaster relief rather than the mass trauma circumstances that are more likely in large-scale combat operations. Mass trauma is not routinely practiced as it was during the Cold War. This could indicate an opportunity for the timely reintroduction of triage training at MTFs and during exercises similar to the Medical Red Flag events regularly held in the 1980s.[11]

Using Autonomous Drones for Medical Resupply

As noted, one of the key challenges to large-scale casualty support is ensuring that there are adequate supplies on hand. However, under CDO conditions, it may be problematic to assume consistent availability of delivery platforms to distribute medical resupply packages to MTFs across the combat theater. Consequently, it may be helpful to have access to a variety of transportation platforms. Outside of conflict, other environmental challenges, such as those in the wake of natural disasters, similarly motivate the need for fast, flexible, and resilient resupply options.

Autonomous unmanned aerial vehicles (UAVs), commonly referred to as drones, offer a potential solution. UAVs are employed in the commercial sector for a range of on-demand medical delivery applications. For example, Zipline is a firm that offers autonomous drone delivery services in Rwanda and Ghana, and it began to explore

---

[11] See Thomas L. Sack, "Improved Combat Casualty Medicine," *Air Force Magazine*, August 1, 1981.

opportunities to support military exercises in 2019.[12] Commercial competition in this market has grown as well. Dutch firm TU Delft develops drones to deliver medical equipment to first responders and U.S. company Vayu designs drones that can shuttle medical supplies and samples, just to name two players.[13]

In the context of resupply during combat, medical operations could benefit from access to UAVs. For example, should it prove too hazardous to use ground transportation for medical resupply missions, time-sensitive delivery by an autonomous UAV platform could help offset that risk and meet at least some demand for life-saving supplies. However, the requirements for medical delivery UAVs in combat have not been thoroughly evaluated. Formal assessments will highlight key performance parameters for these platforms, including payload capacity, delivery range, and loiter capability.[14]

The possible introduction of a new transportation asset to the medical domain brings up a range of logistical and organizational questions. Foremost among them is the need to address who will own and operate the systems; the MHS does not currently possess UAV platforms, and formal requirements will need to be devised to guide the acquisition of specific platforms. It is possible that combat units associated with deployed medical support teams will be a natural fit for the operation of resupply drones. However, they will need to be closely synchronized with their medical counterparts to ensure the safe and seamless delivery and handling of medical materiel.

Given the unknowns, there may be an opportunity for contracting support in UAV resupply operations. Augmentation through a contracted logistics capability can enhance this valuable support function while offering the MHS opportunities to assess the trade-offs of

---

[12] Jacob Douglas, "Zipline Testing Medical Supply Drones with US Military," CNBC, October 22, 2019.

[13] Sebastien Roblin, "Will Blood-Bearing Delivery Drones Transform Disaster Relief and Battlefield Medicine?" *Forbes*, October 22, 2019.

[14] The analytic community has developed tools for assessing the tradespace of UAV performance parameters. See, for example, Christopher K. Gilmore, Michael Chaykowsky, and Brent Thomas, *Autonomous Unmanned Aerial Vehicles for Blood Delivery: A UAV Fleet Design Tool and Case Study*, Santa Monica, Calif.: RAND Corporation, RR-3047-OSD, 2019.

organic military ownership of resupply UAVs. It is important to consider the threat conditions under which contractors would need to operate. For instance, it might be too risky to employ contract support in an active combat environment. In contrast, contracting may prove more viable in exercise settings or in day-to-day operations across the steady-state MTF network.[15]

The question of system ownership and operation drives another key consideration—namely, how UAV platforms would be maintained and by whom. The MHS would need to consider whether members of the medical community would need to plan for and conduct UAV maintenance. If this key sustainment function were to be supported by other functional specialties currently performing UAV maintenance, such as drone operators (including contracted maintenance support), these crews will likely need to operate in close coordination with the medical teams they support. For example, maintainers benefit from a detailed understanding of planned requirements in terms of the number of available platforms and their expected sortie rates. These factors help in estimating the size of the maintenance force and any requirements for spare parts and drone subassemblies.

Another fundamental issue is how drone operators would be trained to use autonomous delivery platforms. The MHS does not currently train any staff in flight procedures or airspace management. These skill sets fall outside the traditional domain of the medical community, and it could prove challenging to develop and to ensure continuity of skills among those selected to operate resupply UAVs. In similar fashion, it will be important to establish standards and qualification levels for medical supply UAV operators to guide training and certification processes.[16]

---

[15] This report returns to the question of when it might be most beneficial to contract for logistics support in Chapter Five.

[16] Given the novelty of this potential future mission set for the MHS, it may prove challenging to develop these standards according to a "train as we fight" principle. For more, see Bernard D. Rostker, Charles Nemfakos, Henry A. Leonard, Elliot Axelband, Abby Doll, Kimberly N. Hale, Brian McInnis, Richard Mesic, Daniel Tremblay, Roland J. Yardley, and Stephanie Young, *Building Toward an Unmanned Aircraft System Training Strategy*, Santa Monica, Calif.: RAND Corporation, RR-440-OSD, 2014.

Finally, each of these considerations will come into play in assessing the total costs of ownership of a UAV platform for medical resupply. Procurement, training, and maintenance feed into estimates of both the upfront and recurring costs of drone ownership. In viewing these parameters holistically, MHS senior leadership will be better positioned to assess the future potential to implement this intriguing solution.

Conclusions

This chapter began with the observation that the current paradigm for medical support is limited in the face of conditions expected in future combat operations. Access to quality care could be constrained by three key factors: the capability at MTFs to offer quality care to the wounded, the capacity of field hospitals to treat and hold large numbers of combat casualties, and the ability to expedite patient throughput at MTFs. A number of mitigations could help in one or more of these dimensions, including first responder training; augmenting modular MTFs with increased patient holding capacity, especially in critical care wards; and pairing resilient resupply mechanisms with triage strategies specific to mass trauma events to accelerate patient throughput.

Expeditionary medical facilities will be highly resource-constrained in the face of mass trauma conditions, and attempts to alleviate congestion and improve care with a single mitigation strategy can exacerbate bottlenecks farther along in the network of care. Consequently, the MHS will likely need to take a portfolio approach and select multiple mitigation strategies to improve outcomes for the largest number of combat casualties.

However, the scenarios described in this chapter were predicated on one very essential assumption: that medical materiel and facilities are available in theater prior to the onset of a conflict. The 2018 NDS acknowledges the potential for a rapid onset of hostilities in the future combat environment. Chapter Four addresses this challenge by exploring the mechanisms to ensure that critical medical assets are close at hand and that the military's network of expeditionary MTFs is established before the first combat casualties require treatment.

CHAPTER FOUR

Enhancing the Global MHS Network of Medical Supply Caches

The previous chapter examined how the evolving threat environment could drive larger numbers of casualties in a future conflict than the MHS has needed to treat during combat operations over the past several decades. This increased demand signal for casualty care will likely call for adaptations in how an expeditionary care network is postured to ensure that medical support is readily available to handle these surges. The 2018 NDS also suggests that U.S. forces should prepare to rapidly mobilize for future combat operations. Consequently, the MHS will need to have the necessary capabilities in place to receive patients quickly.

These threats drive another fundamental question: Can the MHS rapidly establish a network of field hospitals across a future combat theater? The bulk of medical equipment and consumable supplies, such as bandages and basic pharmaceuticals, is stored centrally in CONUS facilities. There are several advantages to this strategy in that it leverages economies of scale to keep warehousing, maintenance, and routine inspection costs low.

However, it also means that the assets needed to get military field hospitals up and running a great distance from likely deployment locations. Rapid deployment would require significant airlift support if materiel and supplies are to arrive in theater prior to the initiation of a conflict. Consequently, a natural tension arises between the extra cost of sustaining a global medical warehousing network and the increased speed with which medical assets could be deployed. This chapter discusses the factors that influence decisions about both cost and effectiveness, as well as where assessment and analysis could inform the trade-offs between them.

Medical Materiel Storage Decisions for a CDO Environment

In the weeks leading up to a potential large-scale conflict, the U.S. military would encounter several challenges to rapidly transporting medical assets to the theater. Medical materiel and supplies would compete for transport space with the significant number of military assets that must flow into the theater immediately, including combat vehicles, munitions, and maintenance equipment. These capabilities are important to prioritize in the flow of forces because they can play a key role in deterring an adversary's decision to initiate a conflict. However, their deployment also requires a significant allocation of lift assets. This is especially true for operating locations at great distance from CONUS that the 2018 NDS highlights likely hotspots for future conflict: the Pacific, the Middle East, and Europe.

These combat assets can fully occupy the limited number of airlift platforms for a prolonged period. It would be exceptionally difficult to get additional cargo on board these transports during the critical movement window prior to or immediately following the onset of hostilities. As transport space becomes available, it would then be allocated to remaining combat support functions, and medical assets would be in competition with civil engineering, base support services, and other lower-tier priorities. These constraints on access to lift platforms can challenge efforts to move medical materiel and supplies where they will be needed in time to treat a conflict's first casualties.

Augmenting the volume of medical materiel stored across the globe can accelerate its deployment to intended points of end use. If these items are stored regionally, deployment times can be significantly reduced, and a broad range of intratheater lift platforms, including sealift and trucking, can be leveraged to relieve pressure on a stressed cargo movement network. Moreover, regionally stored supplies can serve a dual purpose if U.S. assistance is needed nearby in peacetime, such as in the aftermath of a natural disaster. Dual-use medical materiel can also support military exercises with regional partners, again enhancing its utility. Both these prospects make hosting regional storage more enticing to partner nations and could even lead to cost-sharing agreements.

In recent years, senior military leadership has publicly commented on the value and importance of a prepositioned posture for war reserve materiel (WRM), especially in its ability to support U.S. responsiveness in short-circuiting an adversary's attempt to limit freedom of movement for U.S. forces in a CDO campaign. In 2015, the head of logistics and mission support for U.S. Air Forces in Europe–Air Forces Africa commented that a rapid military response hinges on the ability to react quickly from within the theater, stating, "The more I can move forward, the less I have to bring with me."[1] Echoing these sentiments, the forces' commander declared, "It's pretty clear we are going to have to go back and start exercising some of the things we used to do in the Cold War."[2] This shift could entail at least a partial restoration of that era's robust U.S. WRM posture in Europe.

The drive to augment prepositioned stocks in theater is not limited to Europe. Military leadership in the Indo-Pacific theater voiced a similar position, remarking on the importance of having "the right supply at the right place for the right reason."[3] Furthermore, by prepositioning dual-use medical materiel, a WRM posture can help reassure regional partners of the U.S. commitment to the region. As noted earlier, reassurance can stem from the awareness that, with an in-theater supply of medical materiel, the United States could provide rapid and robust support during a disaster response operation. These assets can also help deter potential adversary action in the region by projecting

---

[1]   Brig Gen Bradley Spacy, quoted in Marc V. Schanz, "Infrastructure Improvements Key to Engagement," *Air Force Magazine*, July 9, 2015.

[2]   Gen Frank Gorenc, quoted in Marc V. Schanz, "Hardening, Dispersal, and Survivability in Europe," *Air Force Magazine*, September 15, 2015.

[3]   Gen Lori Robinson, commander, Pacific Air Forces and air component commander, U.S. Pacific Command, quoted in Jennifer Hlad, "Right Supplies, Right Place," *Air Force Magazine*, March 1, 2016.

a message that the United States can expedite the deployment of key materiel and respond to regional threats quickly.

Considering Trade-Offs in the Forward Storage of Medical WRM

Given that the topic of prepositioning is of such interest to senior military leadership, it is worth exploring the tradespace of cost and capability in expanding the WRM posture, with a focus on medical materiel.[4] This section examines the core issues underpinning the expansion of prepositioned medical materiel, including the pros and cons outlined in Table 4.1. Why are medical assets an especially useful component of a regional WRM network? In particular, what medical materiel should be prepositioned? Where should it be stored, and how can it be maintained at regional facilities? And how quickly can it be deployed when it is needed?

In essence, what Table 4.1 indicates is that placing medical WRM in or near a theater of interest can offer a number of benefits, namely, the ability to rapidly support contingencies in both peace- and wartime, while freeing up capacity in a stressed long-distance military transportation network. However, this improvement in readiness could come at a cost: More warehouses might be needed for storage in the theater, and additional materiel and manpower might be required to sustain the in-theater WRM network. Understanding the trade-offs between WRM's capability to support rapid deployment and the costs required to sustain a storage network will help senior leaders make

---

[4] Although analysts have examined WRM postures, little attention has been dedicated to the prepositioning of medical materiel. For related assessments of prepositioning asset classes, such as bare base systems and vehicles stored in WRM, see Mahyar A. Amouzegar, Robert S. Tripp, Ronald G. McGarvey, Edward W. Chan, and Charles Robert Roll, Jr., *Supporting Air and Space Expeditionary Forces: Analysis of Combat Support Basing Options*, Santa Monica, Calif.: RAND Corporation, MG-261-AF, 2004, and Ronald G. McGarvey, Robert S. Tripp, Rachel Rue, Thomas Lang, Jerry M. Sollinger, Whitney A. Conner, and Louis Luangkesorn, *Global Combat Support Basing: Robust Prepositioning Strategies for Air Force War Reserve Materiel*, Santa Monica, Calif.: RAND Corporation, MG-902-AF, 2010.

Table 4.1
Pros and Cons of Prepositioning Medical WRM

Pro	Con
Facilitates agile response to contingencies	May need to purchase additional supply to augment prepositioned stocks
Enables deployment by intratheater transport	Requires good relationships with host nations for access to prepositioned stock
Reduces deployment costs	Costs may increase with loss of maintenance economies of scale at currently centralized storage facilities
Frees up intertheater transport to move other assets	Introduces potential throughput challenges at in-theater truck-loading docks and seaports

informed choices about the ultimate disposition and configuration of a global WRM network.

The remainder of this chapter introduces each of these issues and provides a qualitative assessment of how to balance these pros and cons in designing a medical WRM posture.[5]

The Dual-Use Proposition for Prepositioning Medical Materiel

So far, the discussion has offered a broad rationale for prepositioning supplies and equipment across a global network and provided an introductory argument as to the value of storing medical assets in theater, with a focus on its dual role in supporting U.S. and partner interests during peacetime and in conflict operations. This section further assesses the value —and, potentially, the necessity—of prepositioning medical materiel as part of a global WRM network.

---

[5] Appendix B describes a methodology and modeling framework that integrates key constraints and features of the WRM storage and distribution network.

Medical WRM for Supporting Contingencies

In the buildup to conflict operations, the U.S. military follows a carefully scripted plan for deploying assets into the combat theater. This script, known as time-phased force and deployment data (TPFDD), provides a day-by-day deployment schedule of assets that need to flow from their home station to their operational location. The timeline represented in a TPFDD assimilates the movement of assets ranging from high-end combat capabilities to the many assets that support them. Each asset, whether manpower or materiel, is assigned a transportation mode, such as airlift or sealift, and each receives a sequencing order in the overall deployment timeline for its movement into the theater.

TPFDDs supporting conflict operations are carefully designed and sequenced with intended operational effects. For example, offensive and defensive aircraft and crews are often flowed into the theater first to generate a deterrence effect. These assets can signal to a potential adversary that the United States is prepared and committed to defending its interests. Materiel that provides direct support to these aircraft and their missions, such as munitions and maintenance assets, generally follow close behind. Other support is generally unable to flow into the theater simultaneously, given the limited number of transportation assets available to move such a high volume of material and manpower.

Consequently, many other support functions in the remaining logistics tail must compete for priority in the TPFDD. These functions, collectively known as *agile combat support*, span a wide range of capabilities, such as medical support, fuels, security forces, civil engineering, food services, and communications. With the limited throughput available by sealift and airlift, TPFDD planners must consider each function's role and requirements, particularly with respect to supporting the warfight. With a clear understanding of the context for the agile combat support functions, planners are better able to schedule the movement of materiel.

Case Study: Transporting Air Force Medical Materiel for Wartime Support

Assessing and calculating transportation requirements can prove especially challenging if the points of end use for assets are far away from the points of origin at their home stations. In its storage of medical materiel, the Air Force manages this complexity to some degree by maintaining its primary storage points at a relatively small number of larger hubs. The largest warehousing facility is located centrally in CONUS at Kelly Field in San Antonio, Texas.[6] The Air Force also operates key storage points on each coast. These two facilities are at Travis Air Force Base outside Sacramento, California, and Charleston Air Force Base in South Carolina. With this placement of facilities, the Air Force moves assets to the east, west, or south by drawing on available stock from the closest warehouse. The delivery of some assets can also be expedited, given that the Air Force maintains a network of storage points for medical materiel around the globe, although it is relatively sparse.

With respect to medical assets in a TPFDD, one of the most common elements is a suite of materiel and supplies to set up expeditionary MTFs. As highlighted earlier in Chapter Three, the Air Force's deployable field hospitals are collectively known as the EMEDS system, a capability that can be readily scaled to support air base populations of various sizes. The smallest EMEDS package includes room for four patients, as well as a basic emergency room, operating room, and intensive care unit. Larger EMEDS facilities can hold 25 patients and are able to support them with a wider array of medical interventions, such as more-specialized surgical care, and ancillary services, including physical therapy.[7]

Should combat operations initiate prior to the arrival of an EMEDS package, operating locations will need to provide care with

---

[6] As a point of reference, the distance from Kelly Field to Yokota Air Base, a main air mobility hub in the western Pacific, is 6,500 miles, with a nonstop flight time of more than 13 hours.

[7] The common nomenclature for these MTFs is EMEDS+X, where X represents the bed capacity of the facility. Hence, the 25-bed facility described here is known as the EMEDS+25.

the limited medical assemblages, personnel, and supplies on hand. In general, this will entail the small medical capability that can travel with Air Force flying units. The modest level of care that supports flying squadrons is known as an air transportable clinic. This very small facility is staffed by a squadron medical element, which consists of a flight surgeon and two aerospace medicine technicians. The clinic has a limited capacity of three beds, and it is not designed for long-term medical care or to serve mass casualties.

In sum, should hostilities initiate sooner than accounted for in the TPFDD, the higher-capacity and more-robust capabilities offered by EMEDS may arrive too late.

Medical WRM for Support During Peacetime

An additional benefit of prepositioned medical materiel is the accelerated response that the United States can provide in support of humanitarian assistance/disaster relief (HADR) operations. The U.S. military has a long history of supporting HADR, especially in the Indo-Pacific region. Recent operations include assistance to the victims of the 2015 Nepal earthquake (Operation Sahayogi Haat), Typhoon Haiyan in the Philippines (Operation Damayan, in 2013), the 2011 earthquake and tsunami in Japan (Operation Tomodachi), and the 2004 tsunami in the Indian Ocean (Operation Unified Assistance).

Each operation faced challenges. In lessons learned from these operations, U.S. planners noted that they could have benefited from a larger prepositioning posture of medical materiel and MTFs in the Indo-Pacific.[8] To prevent these types of shortfalls in the future, it may be possible to establish agreements to store medical WRM within a partner's borders with the understanding that the partner would directly benefit from these supplies during HADR operations. Should the United States be willing to grant right of first use of these supplies to the partner nation during HADR, it may be possible to

---

[8] Analysts have noted additional ways to improve response, such as exercising HADR scenarios and ensuring that personnel are trained for disaster response and coordination. For more, see Jennifer D. P. Moroney, Stephanie Pezard, Laurel E. Miller, Jeffrey Engstrom, and Abby Doll, *Lessons from Department of Defense Disaster Relief Efforts in the Asia-Pacific Region*, Santa Monica, Calif.: RAND Corporation, RR-146-OSD, 2013.

obtain cost-sharing agreements for their storage and upkeep. For example, in such an arrangement, the partner nation might offer to pay for the lease on warehouse space while the United States provides the medical materiel.

Prepositioned medical assets can also enhance support for exercises and theater engagement events. For example, during Cope North 15, a joint and multilateral exercise held in the area around Guam, the Northern Mariana Islands, and Micronesia in February 2015, an EMEDS package was deployed to Rota in the Commonwealth of the Northern Mariana Islands from Andersen Air Force Base on Guam. The deployment was exercised as a means to simulate support to a population of disaster victims.[9] This allowed the multilateral participants to practice deployment operations and to collaborate in a demonstration of expeditionary medical capabilities. Whether in an exercise or conflict scenario, prepositioned WRM can play a role in the exhibition of international cooperation and cementing regional partnerships.

Thus far, this chapter has illustrated the range of benefits from prepositioning medical assets as part of an overall WRM posture for use in peace- and wartime. Placing medical assets, such as MTFs and key medical supplies, closer to their expected points of end use can promote agility and expedite deployment (and eventual employment) by reducing the timelines that would otherwise be required to transport these assets from CONUS. Furthermore, demonstrating such capabilities as the rapid deployment of MTFs in peacetime can signal the readiness of the U.S. military to counter potential adversary action and shape the regional security environment.[10] With this credible support for the value of prepositioning, the next section turns to an examination of potential candidate assets for forward storage as medical WRM.

---

[9] Melissa B. White, "Natural Disaster Response Improved at Cope North 15," U.S. Air Force, February 23, 2015.

[10] In the current parlance of joint operations planning, this is also known as sustaining operations in Phase 0. As described here, medical WRM may be an asset in preventing a transition to Phase I, deterring adversaries from actions that could escalate to conflict operations. For more on these constructs, see Joint Publication 5-0, *Joint Planning*, Washington, D.C.: U.S. Joint Chiefs of Staff, June 16, 2017.

Evaluating Candidate Medical WRM Assets

Medical Prepositioning Across the Joint Force

The U.S. military services are considering augmenting their prepositioned stocks of war materiel around the globe. Each of the joint partners has its own reasons for prepositioning WRM. Consequently, each has established prepositioning sites and service-specific capability sets both for WRM in general and medical materiel in particular. This section provides an overview of the services' respective approaches to prepositioning—how, where, and when they store medical materiel and how they are attempting to adapt their WRM programs to meet new requirements to support operational plans in a resource-constrained environment.

U.S. Army Prepositioned Stock

The Army's primary purpose in prepositioning assets is to reduce the deployment response time of its CONUS-based forces. In a conflict, the Army would be able to sustain its soldiers until maritime supply lines are established. The Army's prepositioning requirements are based on expeditionary requirements and regional operational plans.

The Army's enterprise prepositioning posture focuses primarily on four sets of land-based Army prepositioned stocks. These stocks are located in CONUS, Europe, Southwest Asia, and the Pacific, with afloat capabilities aboard ships around the globe. As part of this system, the Army stores a robust set of medical capabilities (more broadly known as Class VIII materiel), which is intended to ensure enough initial medical operating capability and follow-on requirements. Representative materiel here may include combat support hospitals and minimal care detachments, as well as their sustainment stocks.[11] Finally, the Army's Office of the Surgeon General organizes the contingency stocks of perishable materiel separately from assets stored with its prepositioned stocks. The Army stores this class of medical consumables

---

[11] A fully developed CSH is a 248-bed facility. A CSH provides a robust suite of medical capabilities similar to that found at a theater hospital. In comparison, minimal care detachments have 120 beds and offer minimal nursing care or rehabilitative services.

(also known as *potency and dated materiel*) in bundles called unit-deployed packages.[12]

U.S. Marine Corps Prepositioning Squadrons Afloat

While the Marine Corps has one land-based prepositioning site located in Norway, its forces in the Indo-Pacific are more dependent on its afloat component, the Maritime Prepositioning Force. A maritime prepositioning ship squadron is intended to provide support to a single Marine expeditionary brigade (MEB). The squadron's capability sets depend on the specific requirements of the Marine Air-Ground Task Force. In terms of medical capabilities, these sets are centrally issued as authorized medical and dental allowance lists. These sets are designed to support a MEB for 30 days and are configured holistically as integral modules; the Marine Corps does not issue any of the contained equipment or supplies separately as individual line items. Only perishable supplies, such as pharmaceuticals and batteries, are maintained as line items, which makes stock rotation more efficient.

In terms of medical treatment capabilities, each squadron includes one 150-bed medical treatment facility with care comparable to that of a Role 3 theater hospital. Should assets need to deploy to land, MPS cargo stores can be discharged pierside within three days or shuttled to shore afloat (as process known as tendering "in stream") within five days. When a MEB is deployed during a contingency, Class VIII assets are held aboard and available for employment. However, if a MEB is not deployed, medical assets from the squadron must be requested and approved by the owning service, the combatant commander, and the Joint Chiefs of Staff.[13]

---

[12] The Army's Medical Potency and Date program for perishable medical consumables is intended to provide sufficient supplies for a unit for the first 31 days of contingency operations (ranging from HADR to a major combat operation), at which time resupply can be provided by war reserve stock and the industrial base. See Adam C. Resnick, Kathryn Connor, Anna Jean Wirth, and Eric DuBois, *Optimizing Army Medical Materiel Strategy*, Santa Monica, Calif.: RAND Corporation, RR-2646-A, 2019.

[13] U.S. Marine Corps, *Marine Corps Class VIIIA Handbook*, Washington, D.C., NAVMC 4000.2A, June 23, 2017.

U.S. Navy Expeditionary Medical Facilities

The Navy has the smallest prepositioning program of all the services due to its expeditionary nature. Its afloat prepositioning is intended to place equipment and supplies aboard ships in key ocean areas to ensure rapid asset availability during a major theater war, HADR operation, or other contingency. Much like the Marine Corps, the Navy provides life-support facilities aboard each maritime prepositioning ship squadron. The Navy is responsible for maintaining the outfitting for these medical facilities, but this does not include prepositioning Class VIII medical supplies with a short shelf life as WRM aboard its vessels. Instead, these supplies are maintained in inventory accounts under a partnership with the U.S. Department of Health and Human Services.

Much as the Army is exploring avenues for leaning deployable medical capabilities, the Navy is examining ways to transform its assets. In 2012, the Navy initiated a plan to upgrade and modernize critical components of its prepositioning program. In part, the program seeks to transform the Navy's larger fleet hospitals, such as the *Comfort* and the *Mercy*, to be more expeditionary in nature.[14]

U.S. Air Force Medical Prepositioning

The Air Force maintains a number of storage sites, both within CONUS and at prepositioning locations around the globe. The assets stored at each location type span the spectrum of Air Force expeditionary medical capabilities: MTFs, medical resupply kits, patient staging systems, collective protection assemblages for use in environments with chemical or biological contaminants, and specialty team equipment sets, such as those used by special forces medical elements.[15]

In general, the assets stored in theater are positioned to support the core functions executed by medical personnel at that base.

---

[14] For more background on the specifics of the transformation initiative, see U.S. Department of Defense, *Report on the Status of Department of Defense Programs for Prepositioning of Materiel and Equipment*, Washington, D.C., 2014. The department produces this regular report to Congress as required by Section 352 of the National Defense Authorization Act for Fiscal Year 2008.

[15] Unique to the Air Force is the en route patient staging system, a deployable facility used for holding patients prior to their aeromedical evacuation to higher echelons of care.

For example, operating locations tasked with personnel recovery are most likely to hold special operations medical gear to support their core pararescue mission. Similarly, closer to sites where potential adversaries might employ chemical or biological attacks, operating locations are more likely to store gear for collective protection against these kinds of agents. By storing a broad array of assets at any individual site, the Air Force is capable of quickly sourcing materiel locally in response to any number of events, ranging from peacetime exercise support to HADR to conflict operations.

However, the in-theater stockage level of any given capability or assemblage is typically not substantial. Consequently, on their own, the forward-positioned stores of medical materiel may be insufficient to fully support a large-scale conflict in a region. Where shortfalls might exist, in-theater shortfalls can be mitigated by flowing assets from the key sites in CONUS to support deployment requirements, as discussed earlier.

DoD's Direction for Joint Prepositioning in WRM

It is clear that each service takes a slightly different approach to the forward storage of its medical assets, assemblages, and supplies. These prepositioning postures depend significantly on the roles each service plays in both conflict and peacetime environments. Moreover, the materiel stored is closely linked with the core medical capabilities that each service provides, based on its fundamental mission sets. That said, the services are making some effort to approach WRM jointly. DoD cautions that this will be a long-term effort, undertaken deliberately and judiciously, and that it will focus its energies on supporting national security objectives by enabling combatant commanders' operations plans and strategic goals. Guidance from the Joint Chiefs of Staff on WRM, released in January 2020, offers a constructive framework, with the stated goal "to achieve an efficient, coordinated, and agile materiel response" to support global combatant commander needs across the range of military activities. The framework helps reduce risk in supporting those plans while limiting the potential for duplication of effort across the military services.[16]

Selecting Storage Sites for Medical WRM

With the underpinnings of why and what to store, the logical next step in this discussion is where to preposition medical WRM. Careful site selection is essential to maintaining equilibrium among many key support factors, such as the network's ability to efficiently deliver stored materiel to the points of end use, the shipment times required for the materiel to arrive at these destinations, and the storage costs at each WRM storage site. The following case study involving WRM storage sites in the Middle East illustrates the importance of site selection and how evolving constraints in operating conditions can drive shifts in site utilization.

Case Study: Medical WRM in U.S. Air Forces Central Command

Thumrait Air Base is situated close to the Arabian Sea in Oman. Thumrait is convenient to other operating locations in the region, such as Al Dhafra Air Base in the United Arab Emirates, Al Udeid in Qatar, and Isa Air Base in Bahrain.[17] Moreover, because Thumrait is an active military site, asset safety is maintained by the base's security forces. Thumrait's WRM stores contain a range of assets, including medical materiel, fuel dispersal hardware, and munitions. Figure 4.1 shows a satellite image of this operating location. The WRM storage site appears in the upper right of the photo, with access to cargo offload/onload pads visible between the main runway and the WRM campus.

During Operation Desert Shield/Desert Storm, the Air Force flew combat missions from Thumrait and used the base to preposition WRM to support TPFDD force flow. Although base was con-

---

[16] Chairman of the Joint Chiefs of Staff Instruction 4310.01E, *Logistics Planning Guidance for Pre-Positioned War Reserve Materiel*, Washington, D.C., January 13, 2020, p. A-2.

[17] Flight distances from Thumrait Air Base to these operating locations are 500–750 miles, with typical nonstop flight times of 1.5 to two hours.

Figure 4.1
WRM Storage at Thumrait Air Base, Oman, in 2020

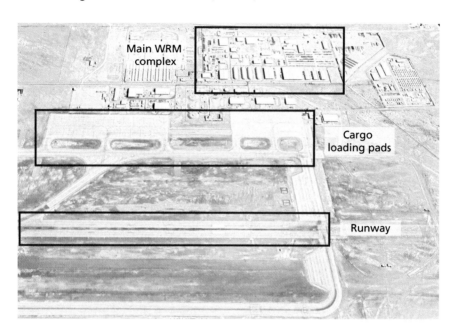

SOURCE: Google Earth.

veniently located in the theater of operations, challenges nevertheless arose in relying on it as a site for both mobility and combat operations. Aircraft throughput was limited by competition for airfield resources, such as fuel hydrants and spaces to park aircraft. Additionally, the staging areas for the onload and offload of cargo frequently became congested, which made it challenging to efficiently support throughput of mobility assets.

To help alleviate the problem, the United States contracted with the commercial firm Maersk at the nearby Omani port of Salalah to support a second WRM site. At Salalah, Maersk was able to provide agile throughput of containerized cargo by onloading and offloading sealift assets. When needed, materiel could be delivered between Thumrait and the port via 50-mile drayage using truck transport.

Maersk was also able to provide asset security at the port.[18] Thus, the U.S. military was able to introduce civilian contract support at an alternative location to not only add a storage point beyond an existing air base but also to free up military security personnel and provide alternative modes of transportation for WRM assets.[19]

Siting Medical WRM

These observations from WRM storage in the Middle East highlight an important feature of site selection for warehouses. Namely, flexibility in transportation options can be an important factor in adapting to evolving constraints. By leveraging access to overland transport, afloat cargo movement, and air cargo platforms, a portfolio of transport options can be called on dynamically in times of need.

It is worth noting that the power of maintaining flexible cargo movement options is not restricted to the Middle East; the same principle applies readily to the Indo-Pacific and Europe. Existing air bases in the region will play a key role in the U.S. military's ability to store, secure, and rapidly move critical assets. In addition, local options for storing medical materiel at partner-nation warehouses may be attractive to some partners, especially if those nations are granted agreements to access these assets to support HADR operations. Cost-sharing arrangements could also be made wherein the partner might agree to pay warehouse leasing or security costs to support the storage of materiel. It might also be possible to work with allies in the region to secure storage options at existing allied operating locations, where

---

[18] It is important to note that sensitive assets, such as munitions, were not stored at Salalah. Such materiel was excluded from storage at the commercial port for both security and safety reasons.

[19] The United States has a strong political relationship with Oman, which underpins the assumption that the United States would have continuing access to such sites as Thumrait and Salalah. In assessing the viability of new or alternative WRM sites, the caliber of political ties with the partner nation should be explicitly considered. See Kristin F. Lynch, Anthony DeCicco, Bart E. Bennett, John G. Drew, Amanda Kadlec, Vikram Kilambi, Kurt Klein, James A. Leftwich, Miriam E. Marlier, Ronald G. McGarvey, Patrick Mills, Theo Milonopoulos, Robert S. Tripp, and Anna Jean Wirth, *Analysis of Global Management of Air Force War Reserve Materiel to Support Operations in Contested and Degraded Environments*, Santa Monica, Calif., RAND Corporation, RR-3081-AF, 2021.

warehouse space may already be available and where security could be provided by the host nation's military forces.

The Middle East case study also demonstrates that commercial partnerships can offer important opportunities to extend the reach and effectiveness of a regional WRM posture. In storing non-provocative and relatively inexpensive materiel for expeditionary MTFs and associated medical supplies at commercial warehouses and port facilities, the U.S. military would be able to expand its reach to a broader array of maritime and overland routes. For example, in the Indo-Pacific region, such storage sites might include the ports of Tokyo in Japan and Subic Bay in the central Luzon region of the Philippines. The next section explores how augmenting a set of storage sites to facilitate access to such multimodal transportation hubs can provide a more robust and cost-effective portfolio of options to enable cargo movement.

Deploying Assets from Medical Storage Sites

The previous section examined the importance of considering and utilizing WRM storage opportunities at an array of potential locations. The resulting collection of storage sites will ideally give planners and logisticians access to a range of options—sea, air, and land—to help to ensure that there are multiple alternatives should the need arise to deploy WRM. This section explores some of the fundamental properties of transportation modalities and how the ability to tap into a robust portfolio of transport options can enhance critical bandwidth and resiliency during deployments.

Cost-Effectiveness of Transportation Modes

As noted earlier, it is important for planners to examine transport options across the spectrum of sea, air, and land assets. Relying on only one transit modality can lead to congestion at individual sites, limiting throughput and hindering the effectiveness of intratheater deployment. However, it is also essential to note that each option offers different strengths and weaknesses in terms of its daily range, throughput capacity, cost, and availability in a given theater.

For example, sealift can offer substantial throughput capacity in terms of the weight and volume it can move, and it does so cost-effectively. However, the slower speeds of afloat assets, such as container ships, can be a barrier in delivering time-sensitive materiel. On the other hand, airlift is very rapid, but this comes at a considerably higher cost and limited cargo capacity. Overland transit, including line-haul trucking, can strike a balance between airlift and sealift. It offers a price point between that of sealift and airlift, and its cargo throughput can be competitive with a sizable trucking fleet.[20] However, access to points of end use from a given WRM storage site may be significantly constrained by regional geography, such as between island-based operating locations in the Indo-Pacific region.

Alternative Transportation Options

This chapter discussed common cargo modalities, but it is important to note that the roster is not exhaustive. In fact, significant, cost-effective overland throughput can be achieved in some regions by rail. For example, Yokota Air Base is a large air mobility hub in the Fussa region of the Tokyo metropolitan area. Yokota is situated very close to a rail hub, and logisticians may be able to tap into that network for delivery to many other potential operating locations on Honshu, Japan's main island. Although rail transit links are not uniformly available across the Pacific theater, where they do exist, they may offer important alternatives for cargo movement.

Alternatives to container ships and large, medium-speed, roll-on/roll-off vessels can provide niche capabilities for sealift. Here, expeditionary fast transport vessels or other wave-piercing catamarans can provide significant lift capability and offer almost twice the speed of a typical container ship. However, these fleet sizes are not large, so the availability of such vessels may be limited, or they might be in very high demand during execution of the TPFDD. Also, in some regions, such as the Philippines and sections of Europe, barge movement could be an option. These vessels can handle significant payloads, but their

---

[20] As a representative example, the Army maintains a large fleet of trucks, and this capacity can be further augmented on the spot market with commercial options.

range and speed are limited. Nonetheless, such capabilities can expand throughput opportunities at favorable cost-capability ratios in the set of cargo transport options.

In addition, other air transport options might be available beyond the fixed-wing assets typically employed. For example, lighter cargo could be moved by drone or sling-loading heavier assets using rotary-lift platforms.[21] Alternative airlift modalities offer varying capabilities and trade-offs in terms of cost versus throughput. However, they can add breadth to the options for delivering cargo to operating locations that might otherwise be difficult to access by road, rail, or sea.

It is worth noting that the need for careful consideration of a portfolio of cargo movement platforms also applies to the movement of patients. Medical planners often rely on air assets to evacuate patients to higher echelons of care. For example, between Role 3 and 4 MTFs, fixed-wing aircraft, such as C-130 and C-17 cargo platforms, are commonly tasked with the patient movement mission. However, if the air fleet is in high demand to move other assets, or if CDO conditions prohibit access to airfields where patients are awaiting transport, it might be necessary to consider patient movement by rail, barge, or other modes.[22]

The Importance of Analytic Assessment in Fleet Selection

Selecting an appropriate and effective transportation fleet can be challenging. Fleet composition will be intimately linked to the site selection for WRM warehouses, and transportation modalities play a critical role in meeting targeted deployment times at attractive cost points. Furthermore, access to individual modalities may be limited by the composition of organic assets in the fleet and the availability of commercial platforms in the region of each warehouse. Consequently, the decisions involved in fleet selection resemble those in portfolio management: Each asset has its own strengths and weaknesses, and it is unlikely that any single element will be the dominant solution. Conse-

---

[21] As noted in Chapter Three, the movement of medical materiel by autonomous drones has become a topic receiving growing attention in recent years. See Gilmore et al., 2019.

[22] Chapter Six further explores challenges in the patient movement mission.

quently, a balanced portfolio of transportation options, in concert with careful selection of WRM sites, will help ensure the timely delivery of WRM assets to their points of end use in a cost-effective manner.

Conclusions

As discussed in this chapter, future combat operations envisioned in the 2018 NDS could not only be large-scale in nature, but they could also initiate rapidly. This combination suggests that the military could be required to treat casualties on the battlefield at scale—and concurrent with the onset of hostilities. Consequently, it is becoming increasingly important for medical planners to ensure that MTFs and expeditionary care networks can be established without delay.

Military planners during the Cold War recognized this possibility as well, driving the development of a robust WRM network in Europe to ensure that needed capability could be set up in the field quickly. Given that robust WRM postures have languished in the intervening years, medical planners will likely need to consider a range of options to reinvigorate the U.S. military's global medical warehousing network. As noted here, a number of important factors come into play, including what to store, where to warehouse it, and how to move it to likely points of end use. Assessment is key to understanding the cost-effectiveness of sustaining the network, and that will require identifying metrics to track network effectiveness, such as the speed with which assets can be issued and transported to their intended points of end use.

The discussion so far has focused on the medical materiel that is important to supporting combat casualties, where it might be best located, and the means for transporting it to operating locations. The next chapter advances the range of related considerations, extending the discussion to topics related to ensuring the resilience and availability of logistics support across the network of expeditionary care.

CHAPTER FIVE

Improving the Resilience of Medical Logistics and Sustainment

So far, this report has addressed many core elements of expeditionary care cost and capability in a future conflict. The evolving threat environment is driving a fresh look at the likely growing requirement for combat casualty care. Medical support could be taxed in the tripartite domains of capability, capacity, and throughput. Furthermore, the risk of rapid initiation of large-scale combat operations is making it more urgent than ever to reconsider how the U.S. military prepositions medical assets to ensure that care is available prior to the first wave of casualties.

With the focus on scaling and adapting medical support, planners and logisticians are facing a new fundamental question: Do medical logistics and sustainment support capabilities warrant a fresh look as well? The question seems germane, especially in light of growing capability requirements to support an expanded medical WRM network. Moreover, medical logistics and sustainment act as crucial enablers of medical support in the combat environment. If the operational tempo for medical care accelerates, logistics requirements will do so as well. This chapter addresses several topics in this domain, beginning with the range of considerations for maintaining medical assets, both in WRM stockpiles and at actively operating MTFs.

Maintaining Medical Materiel

As with any materiel, medical assets on the shelf need to be examined on a regular schedule to determine their current state and operational condition. For example, in WRM stores, tentage needs to be examined for wear, expiration dates need to be checked and pharmaceuticals need to be replaced, and power generators need to be turned on periodically to assess their operability. When it comes to materiel in use at operational MTFs, medical equipment must be maintained, and medical supplies must be ordered as stocks are consumed. Costs are introduced not only in the repair and replacement of assets but also in the provision of manpower to conduct the inspections, make any necessary repairs, and reorder consumed goods.

Constructs for Asset Maintenance

As a starting point, this chapter explores an array of constructs for maintaining medical materiel. The concepts explored here range from those commonly used in the storage and maintenance of medical assets and assemblages to others are paradigms more commonly found in the support of spare parts for aircraft and engines. Each concept has applicability for medical materiel, but it will be important to assess potential cost reductions or agility-related benefits to the medical logistics enterprise.

On-Site Maintenance

Dedicated on-site teams are, by far, the most common construct for maintaining medical assets. In this paradigm, the size of the maintenance team can be scaled to the size of the medical warehouse being supported. A small warehouse would warrant a team of limited size—say, one member to conduct inspections and to maintain records, another to make equipment repairs, and a third to provide oversight and procure new materiel. In such an operation, there can be diseconomies of scale at smaller storage facilities, in that staff may not be fully tasked in their WRM support roles. On the other hand, maintenance operations at larger warehouses can yield significant economies of scale and maximize their allocated staff time. This generates cost efficiencies in terms of the manpower funding required for upkeep of the materiel in storage.[1]

Traveling Maintenance Teams

Another materiel maintenance paradigm employs a team that travels between work sites. In this case, a maintenance crew is stationed at an operating location with a permanent maintenance capability and a limited on-hand stock of materiel. If the team were to work only at this small facility, it would likely be vastly underutilized. To better capture manpower efficiencies, the team rotates to support a number of other facilities that lack dedicated maintenance crews. As this traveling team visits each site in turn, it conducts any necessary inspections and maintenance. It is somewhat uncommon, but the U.S. military does employ this construct. For example, in supporting its existing medical WRM storage sites in South Korea, the Air Force retains some contract labor positions to inspect and maintain prepositioned medical assets. These contractors, home-stationed at Daegu Air Base, rotate among various medical WRM storage sites on the Korean peninsula.

In this traveling team maintenance construct, the enterprise is able to avoid the "open the door" cost of supporting an on-site maintenance team at each work site. Instead, the traveling team visits multiple locations, achieving a higher manpower utilization rate through its cross-site maintenance and inspection duties. Although this manpower efficiency captures some cost savings, additional costs must be introduced to support temporary duty expenses. Members of the traveling team are provided their base wage at their home station, but they require additional temporary duty funds for their travel and billeting

---

[1] This tradespace is well understood and modeled by the Air Force's aircraft maintenance manpower community. That community uses a tool known as the Logistics Composite Model to assess manpower requirements relative to the workload expected to support sortie generation. For more information on the Logistics Composite Model and various manpower postures, see Ronald G. McGarvey, Manuel J. Carrillo, Douglas C. Cato, Jr., John G. Drew, Thomas Lang, Kristin F. Lynch, Amy L. Maletic, H. G. Massey, James M. Masters, Raymond A. Pyles, Ricardo Sanchez, Jerry M. Sollinger, Brent Thomas, Robert S. Tripp, and Ben D. Van Roo, *Analysis of the Air Force Logistics Enterprise: Evaluation of Global Repair Network Options for Supporting the F-16 and KC-135*, Santa Monica, Calif.: RAND Corporation, MG-872-AF, 2009.

while visiting remote facilities. Hence, there is likely to be a balance between team size and the number and size of remote warehouses that each team can support. And this balance may shift, depending on local costs in the regions they travel to.

Asset Swap

A third asset maintenance construct, known as "asset swap," can also prove useful. Rather than posturing maintainers at each site across a network, support teams at operating locations are instead staffed by item inspectors. As inspection teams discover equipment in need of repair, they dispatch these items to a central maintenance hub that has a permanent, on-site team of dedicated repair personnel. Upon receipt of an item in need of repair, the hub "swaps" it and sends forward a functional item from local storage. This hub, also known as a centralized intermediate repair facility, can be scaled to support repairs for a large number of operating locations. Doing so can leverage significant economies of scale in terms of maintenance manpower.[2]

As with traveling teams, the cost savings that can be realized by manpower economies of scale must compete with two new costs. First, the system incurs additional costs to support the transportation of materiel to and from the centralized intermediate repair facility. Second, the facility must maintain a pool of on-hand supplies to populate this transportation pipeline and to ensure that authorized stock levels are maintained across the network of operating locations. Thus, it is important to carefully assess which assets are best suited to this model to capture maximum efficiencies across the medical enterprise.

The Role of Civilian Contracts in Maintenance Support

As mentioned earlier, the MHS occasionally takes advantage of maintenance support from the pool of available contract labor. This can

---

[2] Previous analysis has shown the value of this maintenance concept for the repair of such assets as aircraft engines and electronic warfare pods. For more information, see Ronald G. McGarvey, James M. Masters, Louis Luangkesorn, Stephen Sheehy, John G. Drew, Robert Kerchner, Ben D. Van Roo, and Charles Robert Roll, Jr., *Supporting Air and Space Expeditionary Forces: Analysis of CONUS Centralized Intermediate Repair Facilities*, Santa Monica, Calif.: RAND Corporation, MG-418-AF, 2008.

offer significant savings and agility in asset maintenance, depending on the items supported and the types of tasks that need to be conducted in the upkeep of medical assets. Previous analysis has developed a framework for assessing the value of issuing a contract to the civilian labor force over a reliance on the organic military labor pool.[3] This methodology can help identify the most cost-effective labor-sourcing options for an enterprise's tasks based on two criteria:[4]

1. Is the skill set needed to perform this task unique or otherwise specialized within the MHS enterprise, or are these skills commonly available in the open marketplace? This defines the task's *specificity.*
2. Is the task to be performed a common occurrence, or is it uncommon within the MHS? This determines the task's *frequency.*

Once the specificity and frequency are known, the labor sourcing for performing the task can be assessed using the generalized framework depicted in Figure 5.1. The framework outlines four key sourcing opportunities, generating two options apiece based on the frequency of the task to be conducted.

Sourcing Labor for Infrequent Tasks

For tasks that occur infrequently, there can be little cost advantage for developing a talent pool within the military. For example, the enterprise would likely need to develop a training regimen for developing and supporting the necessary skills within the organic military labor force. Furthermore, sustaining these necessary skill sets organically will likely prove challenging. How would the enterprise manage personnel

---

[3] This analysis examined sustainment decisions as applied to depot-level aircraft maintenance. Nevertheless, this framework is readily generalizable to the concepts discussed here. See John G. Drew, Ronald G. McGarvey, and Peter Buryk, *Enabling Early Sustainment Decisions: Application to F-35 Depot-Level Maintenance,* Santa Monica, Calif.: RAND Corporation, RR-397-AF, 2013.

[4] For more on the underpinnings of this analysis, see Ronald H. Coase, "The Nature of the Firm," *Economica,* Vol. 4, No. 16, November 1937.

Figure 5.1
A Framework for Assessing Maintenance Manpower Sourcing

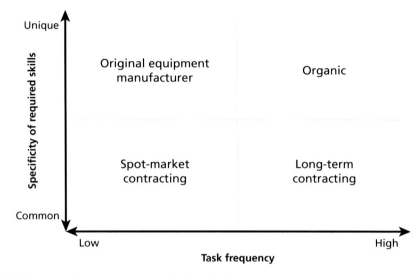

SOURCE: Adapted from Drew et al., 2013, p. 9, Figure 2.2.

with these skill sets, and by what criteria would their promotion and career progression be managed? Consequently, the open market is generally the best option for sourcing labor to perform infrequent tasks.

The taxonomy for labor sourcing outlined in Figure 5.1 breaks down the selection of manpower based on the specificity of the task to be performed. The original equipment manufacturer is likely able to sustain a pool of qualified labor at a meaningful economy of scale and thus could be a cost-effective source of support if a task requires specialized skills. However, should the required tasks rely on more commonly available skill sets, the services could draw on labor obtained through contracts on the spot market. Task commonality should lead to several viable sourcing options in the marketplace, yielding qualified talent at competitive rates.

Sourcing Labor for Frequent Tasks

For tasks that occur more frequently, the enterprise can find opportunities to generate cost effectiveness through economies of scale, looking both within and outside the organic workforce. The decision to insource or outsource can be challenging and depends on a range of factors. Nevertheless, the cost-effectiveness of an option is generally linked to the specificity of the skills required to perform the desired tasks.

With a commonly found skill set, long-term contracts can be established to support required maintenance actions through a non-military labor force. As indicated earlier, the Air Force uses contract civilian labor in South Korea to fill some of its biomedical equipment technician positions. Biomedical equipment technicians inspect, calibrate, and maintain such assets as video displays, physiological monitors, and radiological systems. These skills can commonly be found in the broader U.S. labor pool, as they are needed to support equipment in civilian hospitals. In Figure 5.1, this hiring protocol would fall into the lower right quadrant of the figure, making it ideal for long-term contracting.

For skills that are more specific to core military medical functions, cost-effective manpower solutions should be sourced from within the enterprise. For example, in the case of personnel who directly support the combat medical mission, civilian labor sourcing will not be a viable option in a conflict environment. Some positions might require more security or oversight within the organization, such as staffers who maintain sensitive equipment or manage the supply of controlled pharmaceuticals (e.g., opioids). Increasing task frequency will likely increase the need for qualified personnel who can be sourced and managed organically, as the requisite skills may not be found readily or cost-effectively on the open market. Consequently, meaningful economies of scale for the labor pool here can be achieved organically.

Hybrid Sourcing Selections

Even with the broad framework outlined here, manpower choices can prove challenging, especially when cost-effectiveness is not the only factor in the decision. For example, the MHS has an interest in organically supporting such career fields as biomedical equipment technicians, as this talent pool provides essential skills to sustain equipment in a deployed environment. However, civilians and contract labor can provide continuity of knowledge that would otherwise be unavailable at fixed storage sites as active-duty personnel rotate between duty stations. In these circumstances, the MHS takes advantage of a hybrid solution by employing both active-duty and contract personnel.

Applying the Specificity/Frequency Framework to MHS Medical Provider Positions

It is worth taking a moment to note that the framework described here can be applied to a range of contexts. For example, the MHS is working toward consolidating fixed-facility MTFs under the aegis of DHA; these facilities have historically been managed by the services. Consolidation can offer meaningful savings by integrating data systems, combining orders for block buys of medical supplies and equipment, and slimming the management pool that administers the network. Each of these factors is a consequence of expanding the economies of scale available to a larger network. It is only natural that this consolidation might also look for opportunities to enhance cost-effectiveness within the labor pool of MHS medical providers by rebalancing the mix of uniformed military personnel, civilians, and contracted support.

Consider how the framework in Figure 5.1 might apply in this context. Highly specialized medical care might be required infrequently across the beneficiary population. For example, in steady-state operations, demand for niche neurosurgical procedures might arise only at larger MTFs in CONUS, facilities that support a large, diverse beneficiary base. These specialty surgeries (with high skill specificity and low frequency) could be outsourced to civilian providers. Thus, at first blush, it seems reasonable to pivot such positions from the military labor pool to contractors, DoD civilian providers, or the private sector. Should opportunities to civilianize positions appear at scale, the MTF transition might yield regions in the system of care "that will have civilians providing the majority of care to beneficiaries and a slimmed-down uniform staff focusing primarily on operational medicine."[5]

---

[5] Patricia Kime, "Services Turn Focus to Warfighters as DHA Takes over Military Hospitals," *Military.com*, April 3, 2019.

Before pursuing such opportunities on a large scale, it is important to account for a distinctly military consideration: The MHS must continue to employ a sufficient number of medical and support staff in future combat operations. In that domain, an overreliance on civilian labor, resulting in a "slimmed-down uniform staff," could lead to shortfalls in meeting requirements for qualified, deployable medical personnel to provide care to combat casualties. In fact, to retain high-specificity/low-task-frequency medical providers within the military labor pool, it will likely prove beneficial to develop mechanisms, such as civil-military partnerships, to increase the workload of these military personnel. Doing so can offer broader means for them to sustain their currency in critical skill sets.[6] Consequently, the specificity-frequency framework can be meaningfully employed only when underlying requirements for organic military personnel are also considered.

Leveraging Partner-Nation Medical Support

Thus far, this chapter has discussed the potential utility of leveraging civilian and contract support for medical logistics, noting where opportunities for civilian hires might prove most opportune. With that in mind, a range of jobs will need to be filled by uniformed military personnel, especially positions that will be needed to conduct medical support in a future combat operation.

While thinking through this constrained specificity-frequency process, the MHS might still find that gaps in manning or medical capability could emerge during a contingency. Moreover, as suggested earlier, the demands of large-scale combat operations could also drive shortfalls in the provision of medical logistics and sustainment support. As a means to overcome these potential shortfalls, it may prove advantageous to partner with nations around the world for medical support, with an eye toward securing the availability of critical medical supplies, patient transport, and possibly even treatment for troops wounded in

---

[6]   Steve Sternberg, "A Crack in the Armor: Military Health System Isn't Ready for Battlefield Injuries," *U.S. News and World Report*, October 10, 2019.

combat.[7] Not only might it be an especially relevant mitigation strategy, but it also aligns with the 2018 NDS objective to enhance regional partnerships.

To explore the value of these collaborations for expanding medical support, it can be helpful to consider both the compatibility and capability of regional partners. First, it is important to assess the degree to which each nation shares U.S. security interests to evaluate its likelihood of providing assistance to U.S. forces in a time of conflict. Such assessments should integrate various aspects of compatibility, such as the nation's history of participation in multilateral military operations and exercises with the United States, the alignment of the partner's economic investments and political interests with those of the United States, and its willingness to enter into defense agreements with the United States. An established assessment tool can help visualize the interplay among these dimensions and help identify the relative propensity for cooperation when comparing opportunities with a set of partner nations.[8]

Second, it is equally important to evaluate a candidate partner nation's medical capability, whether relative to the capabilities of a suite of candidate partners or according to a more absolute baseline, such as the medical capabilities available at a Role 3 U.S. MTF. Within the domain of combat casualty care, factors that will be important to assess here will likely include the quality of the nation's blood supply and its standards for testing for pathogens, the standards of care offered at its local medical facilities, and its capacity and capability for patient movement, including medical evacuation by ambulance, helicopter, or fixed-wing aircraft.

---

[7]   Although such partner-nation medical support in combat has not occurred at significant scale in recent decades, it was critical for care to the wounded during World War I. For more, see Emily Mayhew, *Wounded: A New History of the Western Front in World War I*, New York: Oxford University Press, 2014.

[8]   For example, the RAND Security Cooperation Prioritization and Propensity Matching Tool offers these kinds of comparative mapping capabilities. See Christopher Paul, Michael Nixon, Heather Peterson, Beth Grill, and Jessica Yeats, *The RAND Security Cooperation Prioritization and Propensity Matching Tool*, Santa Monica, Calif.: RAND Corporation, TL-112-OSD, 2013.

As shown in the notional map in Figure 5.2, the two dimensions for assessment are a partner's relative propensity for cooperation and the relative quality and capability of the partner's medical support. Depending on where the partner's propensity and capability scores fall, military planners will likely pursue one of three courses of action. For candidate partners whose scores fall near the upper right quadrant of the plot, there may be meaningful opportunities to establish a memorandum of agreement for medical support. These partners could be strong candidates for providing medical supplies or for sharing available hospital capacity in times of international crisis.

Partners whose scores fall toward the center of the plot are more likely to have a modest history of engagement with the United States, as well as a medical capability that falls somewhat short of U.S. standards. One might expect that the partner would benefit from greater assurances of cooperation from the United States, as well as opportunities to

Figure 5.2
Notional Domains of Partner Medical Support in the Propensity-Capability Framework

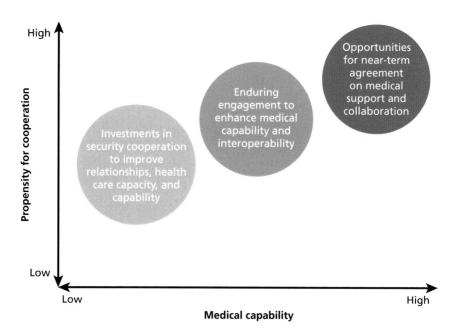

enhance the partner's medical capabilities. Here, interventions to help shift the partner toward the upper right quadrant might include investments to improve the partner's medical evacuation or Role 2 capabilities, as well as routinely conducting bilateral exercises (especially those with a substantive medical component) to increase interoperability and demonstrate U.S. commitment to that partner.

Partners with scores closer to the lower left quadrant will require careful consideration. These nations are more likely to have a limited history of engagement with the United States, and their medical support significantly lags the capability that the U.S. military takes with it into combat. They might also greatly benefit from opportunities to enhance their basic health care, such as through investments in ground ambulance fleets and training to establish a more robust paramedic force. Similarly, the United States could invest in a partner's laboratory testing capabilities to enhance its blood supply safety and quality assurance standards.[9] This type of investment could also foster enduring goodwill and improve U.S. relations with the partner, as this type of capability might improve the quality of life for local populations, in addition to serving as a potential source of support to U.S. forces during contingency operations. Here, it is especially important to consider not only the kinds of capabilities that might help the United States in a time of crisis but also the domains in which the partner would benefit as well.

Case Study: Engaging Partners in the Middle East

As noted, it is important to evaluate each partner's propensity for cooperation with the United States, as well as its medical capabilities. Furthermore, it might be just as important to consider how partners in a region interact with the United States in a support role—and which other partners are likely to participate. Partner nations in the Middle East have a complicated, interwoven history, and the level of support

---

[9]   U.S. Indo-Pacific Command has taken this very approach with three key regional partners: Vietnam, Laos, and Cambodia. The U.S. military launched the Blood Safety Program to enhance testing and to standardize blood donation and banking capabilities with these partners. See U.S. Pacific Command, "Improving Disaster Response Through a Reliable Blood Supply," April 21, 2015.

they might be able or willing to offer the United States during a crisis will be tightly bound to that politico-historical context. In comparison, consider a scenario in which regional partners are unilaterally under existential threat from a common adversary, such as one of the peer or near-peer U.S. competitors highlighted by the 2018 NDS. In this case, partners will be more likely to offer support to the United States because of the mutual risk and potential consequences of an adversary strike.[10]

Similar degrees of nuance in the likelihood of support may appear across a range of contingency activities. Consider a matrix of military actions paired with the partners that might offer support to the United States. Again, the greater the perceived threat to a partner's national security interests, the more likely it may be to offer assistance. To wit, consider a grid such as the one shown in Table 5.1. Individual cells in the matrix could be color-coded according to a partner's propensity for cooperation in each security scenario.

Table 5.1
A Notional Threat-Based Security Cooperation Assessment Tableau

Scenario	Partner							
	Oman	Jordan	United Arab Emirates	Saudi Arabia	Bahrain	Qatar	Kuwait	Other
Force buildup to deter a near-peer adversary								
Response to near-peer adversary first strike								
Response to regional terrorism threat								

---

[10] It is important to note that the extent of support available to U.S. forces will be heavily predicated on the extent to which a partner nation expects casualties among its own military and civilian populations.

An actual assessment framework for a potential conflict would require greater nuance, but Table 5.1 reflects the considerations that would come into play in estimating each partner's propensity for support. During a crisis, however, some regional partners might prove less willing than expected to offer support if specific other partners respond. For example, in a buildup of forces supporting operations to deter impending adversary aggression, Saudi Arabia might be unwilling to expedite support for transnational materiel movements originating from warehouses in Qatar.[11] However, should that threat escalate to full-scale conflict with a shared adversary, the Saudi government might relax its border-transit restrictions.

Expanding this look at partners' propensity to support U.S. operations, there is considerable variation between countries in terms of the medical capabilities they might have to offer. For example, patient movement is likely to be ground-only in smaller countries, whereas larger nations with highly developed economies and militaries will have access to air ambulance services. Countries with the most advanced militaries might have full-scale military medical evacuation capabilities. Even with ground movement, some partners might be able to offer only basic life support ambulance services, while others might have a more robust mix of basic and advanced life support fleets.[12]

Similarly, hospital facilities can be expected to vary considerably by partner, and often within a partner nation. For example, Yemen is unlikely to be able to offer meaningful hospitalization services, given the years of conflict there. In stark contrast, Qatar, Saudi Arabia, and the United Arab Emirates might be able to offer medical support at their hospitals that approaches or meets the standards of U.S. hospitals. Yet, even in these countries there is variability in the quality of hospitals between urban and rural areas. As suggested earlier, however, the

---

[11] Travel restrictions from Qatar apply not only to movement by road but also to the surrounding airspace. See "Qatar Airways Threatens to Sue over 'Illegal' Gulf Blockade," Al Jazeera, July 15, 2020.

[12] Basic life support typically involves an ambulance crewed by emergency medical technicians (EMTs). Care options are extremely limited to little more than patient transport. Advanced life support crews typically consist of both a paramedic and an EMT who provide such services as airway support, cardiac monitoring, and medication administration.

existence of a facility does not guarantee U.S. access. In a small nation under fire—even one with good hospitals—the United States will likely see a severely degraded ability to access those facilities, whether because of limited transport options or because the facility is already at capacity with civilian trauma cases.

Assessing Opportunities and Roles for Partner Nation Medical Support

The case study of partner-nation medical support in the Middle East highlights the diverse challenges that planners and logisticians need to prepare for. To determine how to address these factors, it can be helpful to establish a fundamental assessment framework. Not only can a methodical structure for approaching such a problem aid in identifying opportunities to best leverage partner support, but it can also inform how to most effectively invest in a partner's capability and propensity to help in time of crisis.

At its core, an assessment framework should draw on the three core considerations discussed so far: an evaluation of partner medical capabilities, where there might be gaps in U.S. capability relative to a potential threat, and an assessment of a partner's willingness to contribute support. With these building blocks in mind, a sequential assessment structure seems germane:

- *Appraise the adversary threat* (or threat spectrum). What are the adversary's weapons and their effects, the operating sites and assets most likely to be targets, and the projected number and types of casualties that might occur in an operating location over time?
- *Evaluate medical requirements* to support that casualty population. How many MTFs are needed to treat wounded forces? In tandem, what are the requirements for resupply, evacuation vehicles, and medical providers?
- *Determine where there might be gaps in organic medical support.* Are there enough expeditionary MTFs in service inventories to establish the network of care? Are supply chains agile enough to

provide enough medical materiel to support the casualties? Geographically, where are these gaps located?

- Based on the geographic distribution of potential shortfalls, *identify and assess candidate partner nations.* Among those candidates, which have the greatest propensity to support U.S. forces? Which have adequate capability and capacity to help in the domains in which support is needed? Where might those capabilities help bridge gaps in support, and where might shortfalls still remain?
- From the assessment of candidate partners, *evaluate the mechanisms to incentivize partners that are most interested in working with the United States.* Given a partner's own national security interests, is that nation more interested in U.S. investment to enhance or expand a specific clinical or logistical capability, or is it more vested in improving the interoperability of its existing proficiencies with U.S. capabilities?

Such an analysis can identify where U.S. security interests intersect with the partner's and where the partner might have particular medical capabilities to contribute. This process helps target U.S. security cooperation resources most efficiently and effectively to bolster partners' capabilities, improve their propensity to cooperate, or, ideally, both. Moreover, there might be opportunities to leverage existing security cooperation engagement—for example, by incorporating a medical component into the next annual multilateral military exercise with a partner or group of partners.

On this point, in considering future security cooperation engagements, military planners should endeavor to apply U.S. resources to improve a partner's potential to enhance regional security and interoperability with the United States to meet U.S. national security objectives. At its core, this is a complex problem whose solution requires allocating scarce resources. In the context of medical support, resource investment dollars could support personnel exchange programs, training and equipping to improve a partner's medical capacity, exercises to promote and sustain interoperability, and agreements to support prepositioning. Additional resources could also be used to upgrade or sustain a partner's advanced medical capabilities, such as its capacity to respond to chemical or biological attacks. Just as fundamental to the challenge of incentivizing partners and shoring up their capabilities are decisions about which investments should go toward which partner. If resources were unconstrained, a security cooperation planner might seek to invest in each capability across all partners of interest.

Naturally, the reality of the situation is more complex. The U.S. military lacks enough security cooperation planning personnel, materiel, and funding to engage with every partner in every domain of interest. The bandwidth available to focus on the targeted medical equities discussed here is no exception. Furthermore, funding is insufficient to promote all activities or investments with each partner, even within the tightly defined domain of medical support.

Even if the resources available to U.S. planners were unrestricted, the partners themselves have limited ministerial or administrative staff across their governments' functional domains to integrate large infusions of resources, equipment, or staffing into their day-to-day operations.[13] As noted earlier, an investment with a partner is most likely to achieve its intended strategic aim if that capability aligns with the partner's own national security or health strategy. Thus, the challenge at hand is not so much how many different medical capabilities the United States should invest in. Instead, it is a question of which areas to target to maximize the yield on the strategic investment.

Improving the Situational Awareness of Medical Materiel

Up to this point, the discussion of medical logistics and sustainment has examined a variety of means to manage the upkeep of medical materiel and equipment, mechanisms for how to effectively staff this

---

[13] This available bandwidth to receive external support is often referred to in the security cooperation literature as *absorptive capacity*. For more on targeting resourcing to ensure that absorptive capacity is not exceeded, see Angela O'Mahony, Ilana Blum, Gabriela Armenta, Nicholas Burger, Joshua Mendelsohn, Michael J. McNerney, Steven W. Popper, Jefferson P. Marquis, and Thomas S. Szayna, *Assessing, Monitoring, and Evaluating Army Security Cooperation: A Framework for Implementation*, Santa Monica, Calif.: RAND Corporation, RR-2165-A, 2018.

key workforce, and where partner nations might play a valuable role in bridging gaps in medical logistics capabilities. At this point, it is helpful to take a closer look at a key enabler across this medical logistics enterprise: The ability to maintain awareness over the status of medical materiel being supplied to MTFs, as well as the status of assets and supplies at medical facilities across the network of care. The existing systems that provide SA offer a high level of support under steady-state conditions. However, in the high-intensity conflict scenarios projected by the 2018 NDS, there might be a need to implement mitigation strategies to limit disruptions to SA.

This discussion begins with an overview of the variety of medical logistics data systems that provide SA of medical materiel at MTFs across the network of care. These systems support a variety of logistics functions, from placing orders for medical supplies and materiel to tracking the status and location of medical equipment, depending on the system and the user's level of access. The DHA program that oversees the individual data systems is known as the Defense Medical Logistics–Enterprise Solution (DML-ES). Four of the key systems that fall under the purview of DML-ES are as follows:

- *Defense Medical Logistics Standard Support Customer (DMLSS)*, a system that allows users at WRM storage sites and MTFs to place and manage orders for medical materiel[14]
- *DMLSS Customer Assistance Module (DCAM)*, a laptop-deployable software platform that allows lower-echelon MTFs the capability to order medical materiel from deployed locations[15]
- *Theater Enterprise-Wide Logistics System (TEWLS)*, a platform that allows medical supply officers to track inventory and its loca-

---

[14] Defense Health Agency, "DMLSS: Just-in-Time Logistics," factsheet, Falls Church, Va., February 2018.

[15] Defense Health Agency, "DCAM: Defense Medical Logistics Standard Support Customer Assistance Module," factsheet, Falls Church, Va., October 2020a.

tion within a medical warehouse and facilitates its distribution to end users[16]

- *Joint Medical Asset Repository (JMAR)*, the software system that provides users with SA across the medical logistics enterprise, offering various reporting options that allow users to, for example, monitor the status of inventory by location. JMAR also analyzes historical trends to forecast medical materiel needs.[17]

At the time of this writing, DHA was integrating several of these legacy systems into a more-centralized, web-enabled platform known as LogiCole. Once LogiCole reaches full operational capability, it will supplant three of these legacy systems: DMLSS, TEWLS, and JMAR.[18]

During steady-state operations, the execution of medical logistics tasks tends to proceed smoothly. This is made possible by the free flow of information, ready access to cargo platforms for both air and surface delivery, a responsive supply chain for medical materiel, and access to a global network of medical warehouses. Collectively, these medical logistics enablers help to expedite the medical enterprise's observe-orient-decide-act (OODA) cycle.[19] For example, medical logistics data systems allow a user to take note of current supply levels (observe), evaluate how long that stock will support operations at an MTF (orient), choose among a variety of suppliers for replacement stock (decide), and place an order with a vendor (act). At each stage of the OODA cycle, these systems facilitate feedback loops in the decisionmaking process,

---

[16] Defense Health Agency, "TEWLS: Modern Military Medical Logistics," factsheet, Falls Church, Va., October 2020d. TEWLS is commonly used by staff at larger warehousing facilities, such as U.S. Army Medical Materiel Centers.

[17] Defense Health Agency, "JMAR: Total Asset Medical Visibility," factsheet, Falls Church, Va., October 2020c.

[18] DHA intends to host LogiCole on the Amazon government cloud. As of this writing, LogiCole was expected to reach full operational capability in 2023. Defense Health Agency, "DML-ES/LogiCole: Innovative, Integrated, Intelligent," factsheet, Falls Church, Va., October 2020b.

[19] For more on the framing of the OODA loop concept and its incorporation into military planning and operational processes, see Robert Coram, *Boyd: The Fighter Pilot Who Changed the Art of War*, New York: Hachette Book Group, 2002.

in which information gained during any step in the cycle can be revisited and reconsidered prior to executing the desired action. In sum, the operational effect of quality SA using these platforms is the delivery of medical materiel across a global network that enables medical care across the MHS.

However, during combat, an adversary could exploit opportunities to disrupt these systems. Given that the SA of medical materiel relies on an assortment of data systems and communication networks, an adversary's ultimate choice of target and mode of disruption can yield a range of potential operational effects. For example, a missile attack on a communication node could at least temporarily disable the transmission of orders or U.S. planners' visibility of the medical logistics network. Alternatively, an adversary could launch a cyberattack in an attempt to corrupt data in the medical logistics system. In such a scenario, trained local operators would need to manually identify discrepancies in the data, such as on-hand supply reports and resupply orders. Should system users fail to quickly recognize corrupted data, medical support at an MTF could be delayed until orders of required supplies are delivered. In essence, disruptions to medical data systems have the potential to lengthen MHS OODA loops, degrading the efficiency and effectiveness of logistics support to the network of care.

In a future conflict, missile strikes could generate significant spikes in the need for combat casualty care. Simultaneously, the damage from these strikes can limit throughput and the freedom of movement at key logistics and mobility nodes. As a result, U.S. forces must prepare to operate in a future combat environment with a degraded availability of medical supplies and degraded visibility of the delivery pipeline, along with larger numbers of casualties at the very time those supplies are needed the most.

For this reason, the MHS might consider it worthwhile to evaluate mitigation strategies that increase the resilience of SA of medical supplies and equipment across the enterprise. Medical planners may also need to consider how future conflict conditions could lengthen OODA loops and how these mitigation strategies can help accelerate them in the face of adversary disruption and attack. To this end, the MHS might consider adopting the following strategies:

- *Facilitate access to multiple communication channels* (e.g., fiber, cell, microwave, satellite links). With access to multiple modes of communication, U.S. forces can sustain SA even if one mode goes offline. A portfolio of options would help constitute a PACE (primary, alternate, contingency, and emergency) plan for communications.
- *Evaluate the utility and composition of "push" packages of medical supplies.* Should communication with a forward MTF be cut off, planners might have reason to believe that the operating location is under attack and in need of medical supplies. Given that the MTF is unable to place orders (also known as "pull" logistics), a nearby medical supply warehouse could automatically route a pre-configured package of supplies to the MTF that would be useful in providing trauma care.
- *Expand the network of medical supply caches around the globe.* As discussed in Chapter Four, this would reduce the distance between any given operating location and a site where medical supplies are available.
- *Develop training events in which SA of medical logistics is degraded or lost.* Given that logisticians typically have reliable access to such systems as DMLSS and DCAM, it might be valuable for them to train to operate under conditions of denied or degraded access. Learning objectives could focus on how to employ alternate modes of communication and how to activate other means of requisitioning supplies (e.g., sending paper forms by courier, contingency contracting with local suppliers).

Conclusions

As illustrated in this chapter, medical logistics plays an important role in ensuring that service members have enduring access to medical support. To improve the efficiency and cost-effectiveness of medical logistics, it is beneficial to establish alternative constructs for maintaining medical materiel and staffing the logistics workforce. Additionally, to improve the resilience of medical logistics under the conditions of future combat operations, the MHS could explore options to secure logistics and sustainment support from partner nations. Future conflict conditions could degrade reliable and sustained SA over the medical logistics network, where a range of mitigations may be warranted to maintain access to resupply channels.

Now that this report has explored an array of considerations for enhancing the resilience of medical support to deployed operations, it examines how these same challenges could affect warfighter support much closer to home.

CHAPTER SIX

Preparing Medical Support for Homeland Missions

Up to this point, this report has explored several potential challenges for the MHS in providing combat casualty care at contingency locations abroad. Many of the mitigation approaches discussed thus far are predicated on the difficulties of providing care far from the United States and have included prepositioning medical materiel or establishing agreements for securing partner-nation medical support to accelerate access to medical care and supplies.

In addition to addressing the possibility of threats to U.S. forces at contingency locations around the world, the 2018 NDS also calls out threats far closer to home. What are some possible drivers for medical care in these homeland defense and homeland support missions, and how might they yield additional stressors that the MHS could consider in its planning? This chapter explores some of these scenarios and the challenges they might pose to providing support to wounded service members.

Protecting the Homeland by Defending the Arctic

Of the defense objectives highlighted in the NDS, an essential priority for DoD is to defend the homeland from attack. As noted in Chapter One, adversary efforts to field long-range precision weapon systems complicate this critical mission. Pivotal in the network of operating locations supporting homeland defense is the subset of bases located in arctic and subarctic zones. These locations are geographically well suited for such missions as missile warning, air defense, control of space assets, and personnel recovery in the event of a mass casualty event in the region or a transpolar attack by an adversary.[1] Consequently, in recent years, DoD and the U.S. Department of Homeland Security have been paying increasing attention to the importance and continuity of arctic operations for sustaining the key mission of defending the homeland.[2]

Figure 6.1 helps contextualize the importance of operations in the Arctic, depicting the range of military operating sites in and around the Arctic Circle. Russia operates the largest large number of military installations in the region. The United States manages several bases in Alaska and Greenland. A range of partner nations also support operations in the Arctic, including Canada, Denmark, Iceland, Norway, Sweden, and Finland.

Conducting military operations from these sites can prove challenging in terms of both execution and sustainment due to the region's harsh climate and geographic austerity. If an adversary targeted a military installation in the Arctic with conventional weapon systems, the scarcity of resources and geographic remoteness of these installations would make it difficult to overcome degraded capability or recover from outages or supply disruptions. As a result, any decision to invest in base resilience, both to avoid and to rapidly recover from an attack's damage, must take into account the amount of time and logistical complications involved in sending additional assets from other locations. These issues have been the subject of increasing attention in recent years and are a high priority for DoD leadership.[3]

---

[1] For a specific example of arctic air base operations, see Joanne Castagna, "Thule Air Base, Arctic—Consistently on Top of Its Game," U.S. Army, December 13, 2019.

[2] For more on the recent U.S. government focus on the Arctic, see Abbie Tingstad, *Climate Change and U.S. Security in the Arctic,* testimony presented to the Subcommittee on Transportation and Maritime Security, Committee on Homeland Security, U.S. House of Representatives, Santa Monica, Calif.: RAND Corporation, CT-517, September 19, 2019, and Abbie Tingstad, Stephanie Pezard, and Scott Stephenson, "Will the Breakdown in U.S.-Russia Cooperation Reach the Arctic?" *Inside Sources,* October 12, 2016.

[3] For example, North American Aerospace Defense Command has been hosting symposia related to arctic air power projection. See Canadian North American Aerospace Defense

Figure 6.1
Military Installations in the Arctic Region

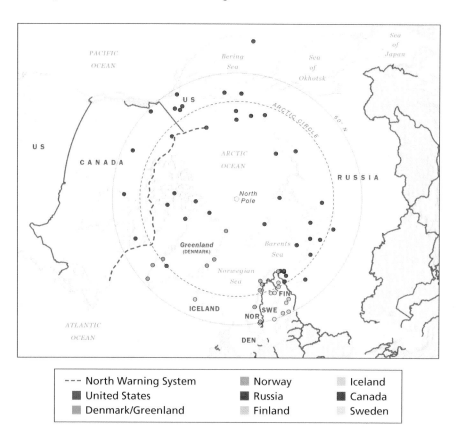

SOURCE: U.S. Department of the Air Force, *Arctic Strategy: Ensuring a Stable Arctic Through Vigilance, Power Projection, Cooperation, and Preparation*, Washington, D.C., July 21, 2020, p. 5.

NOTES: Dots represent selected military operating locations. The dashed line across northern Canada and Alaska represents the early warning radar network used in the air defense of North America.

As part of this growing focus, DoD and the services have begun developing strategic plans for U.S. operations in the Arctic. In tallying risks to domestic security, DoD recognizes that the Arctic is a potential

---

Command Region Public Affairs, "Third Edition of the Arctic Air Power Seminar Welcomes International Experts Leaders, Military Members Alike," February 3, 2020.

vector through which an adversary can strike and that adversary action in the region could degrade the U.S. military's ability to mobilize and deploy forces, materiel, and support around the globe.[4] The Air Force offers one service-level perspective, given its key mission sets in the region: The Arctic is "the keystone from which the U.S. Air and Space Forces exercise vigilance."[5] Consequently, the Air Force has established plans to improve its power-projection capability in the Arctic and is investing in base infrastructure to strengthen resilience, exercises to improve its operability under Arctic conditions, and collaborations with regional partners to enhance deterrence against adversary aggression. In tandem with this growing level of attention from senior military leadership, the MHS will likely prioritize the Arctic in its strategic planning as well.

The sections that follow discuss basic aspects of military operations at an arctic operating location, including medical support, starting with an overview of the challenges stemming from the climate.

Environment and Climate

Arctic and subarctic installations are geographically clustered near or above the Arctic Circle, a latitude of approximately 66 degrees north of the equator. Depending on the location, temperatures in arctic regions can vary tremendously by season, with interior areas seeing temperature swings between 70–80° F in summer and −50° F in winter. Seasonal temperature variations tend to be more moderate in coastal locations, especially where ocean currents, such as the Gulf Stream, provide a buffer against harsher extremes. Similarly, precipitation varies significantly by location. Expected snowfall in Fairbanks, Alaska, for example, is roughly five feet per year, whereas the coastal regions of northwestern Greenland typically see under five inches annually.

Sea ice is a frequent hazard to ship traffic in this region. Afloat shipping may be restricted by season or require icebreaker escorts to

---

[4]   Office of the Under Secretary of Defense for Policy, *Report to Congress: Department of Defense Arctic Strategy*, Washington, D.C., June 2019.

[5]   Quote from then–Secretary of the Air Force Barbara Barrett in U.S. Department of the Air Force, 2020, p. 10.

ensure freedom of access. Surface terrain is typically characterized by permafrost, and this poses a number of challenges to construction and day-to-day operations at military installations. Climate change has led to a thawing of the permafrost in some areas, compromising the integrity of built infrastructure, and has made maritime navigation riskier and less predictable as free-floating sea ice proliferates.

Another factor to account for in the Arctic is seasonal variation in the number of daylight hours. During midsummer (June and July), Arctic locations see 24 hours of daylight. However, during winter (October–March), these same sites are dark nearly round the clock. The limited daylight and extreme cold temperatures can create significant complications for sustainment (e.g., fuel resupply), base construction (e.g., runway repair), and general flight operations in the winter.

Furthermore, the austerity of the Arctic is generally not conducive to supporting large population centers or industrial hubs. There are exceptions to this rule just south of the Arctic Circle, where warmer water currents connect with port regions in Murmansk in Russia and Reykjavik in Iceland, for example. By and large, though, many Arctic sites can expect limited supply chain support in the winter months, except by airlift. Even areas with surface road connections—such as between the subarctic locations of Eielson Air Force Base and neighboring Fairbanks, Alaska—can expect disruptions during challenging winter weather conditions.

It is important to consider the challenges to providing medical support and the implications for combat support functions in the Arctic with these regional characteristics in mind. The following discussion also addresses challenges to these operations if an Arctic installation comes under conventional attack.

Challenges to Medical Support in the Arctic During Steady-State Operations

The austerity of the Arctic's environment and harshness of its climate drive a range of considerations for planning, operating, and sustaining the medical support mission. For steady-state support, a small operating location in a low-threat region typically warrants a limited cohort of medical staff and a small clinic. The medical team for, say, a flying squadron, might consist of only a flight physician and a pair of supporting medical technicians to staff the clinic. Their day-to-day caseload typically involves certifying air crews for flight and providing treatment for minor issues, such as sprains and respiratory ailments. More-serious medical problems will require a patient to be transported to a treatment site off-base that offers more definitive care options. Given the distances that are typical in the Arctic, conditions requiring urgent care will require aeromedical evacuation, as ground ambulance service will likely be too slow, if it is even available at all.

In the Arctic, several medical conditions are uniquely prevalent. Given the extreme cold and very dry environment, clinic staff need to be appropriately trained to receive patients with four categories of conditions: frostbite, hypothermia, dehydration, and, given the local geography, altitude sickness.[6] Even when troops have been issued specialty gear to protect them against extreme cold, such as moisture-wicking layers, vapor barrier boots, and arctic mittens, not wearing the gear consistently or correctly increases the risk of medical conditions related to exposure to the cold.

Medical Materiel and Staffing Challenges in an Austere Environment

The range of trauma injuries resulting from combat operations can rapidly tax the skills and availability of staff at a small clinic. Clinics in austere locations are generally not equipped or staffed to support an operating suite or intensive care unit. Consequently, at a higher-risk operating location, it becomes increasingly important to think through materiel solutions as medical capability augmentation strategies. Recall from earlier discussions how prepositioned medical materiel can offer an important opportunity to rapidly scale up facilities and equipment for medical support. However, on-site storage drives a need for periodic inspections, repairs, and replacement of medical equipment and materiel. Planners will need to weigh the costs and benefits of a dedicated

---

[6] The Army has thoroughly documented a wide range of care requirements in extreme climates. See, for example, Kent B. Pandolf, and Robert E. Burr, eds., *Medical Aspects of Harsh Environments*, Falls Church, Va.: U.S. Army Office of the Surgeon General, 2001.

on-site team or a traveling maintenance team, noting that a traveling team might be able to visit operating locations in the Arctic only during limited windows of time and favorable weather.

Furthermore, in an austere operating location, it is important to take into account the need for medical staff augmentation to populate an Arctic MTF in the event of a conflict. The day-to-day caseload could be inadequate to justify a permanent cadre of specialty staff on site, such as surgeons and critical care nurses, who must maintain the currency of their medical skills, especially those needed to treat combat casualties. However, as discussed, the challenges of transporting such staff to operating locations in the Arctic would only be exacerbated in a conflict scenario.

Special Considerations for Trauma Care in the Arctic

In addition to the special considerations involved in scaling medical support to meet the needs of an operating location under attack, the Arctic poses additional challenges related to caring for trauma patients. These challenges fall broadly into three categories: stabilization, treatment, and evacuation.[7]

In stabilizing a trauma patient in an extremely cold environment, it is important to prepare for the types of injuries they are likely to have. As noted in Chapter Two, in the wake of a conventional attack, casualties are likely to suffer from fragmentation wounds, burns, and injuries resulting in severe hemorrhage. In each of these cases, a patient will require fluids, ranging from lactated Ringer's solution for burns to blood products, such as plasma or red blood cells, for active hemorrhaging.[8] Stabilizing such patients in the Arctic can prove exceptionally challenging because a patient's veins are likely to contract in the cold, and the plastic tubing used for intravenous transfusions can crack and rupture in extremely low temperatures. The climate can

---

[7] Providing treatment to victims of a 1989 C-130 crash in the Arctic demonstrated these three characteristic challenges. See David E. Johnson and W. Bryan Gamble, "Trauma in the Arctic: An Incident Report," *Journal of Trauma*, Vol. 31, No. 10, October 1991.

[8] Sustaining an adequate supply of blood and blood products for trauma patients in the combat environment can be especially challenging, even in the absence of the difficulties the Arctic presents. For more, see Thomas et al., 2018.

also increase the fragility of perishable supplies; for example, lactated Ringer's solution can become unusable in freezing temperatures. Due to rapid fluid loss, in the absence of intravenous fluid replacement or transfusion, patients are at greater risk of hypothermic shock.

Consequently, a key component of cold-weather medical care is getting a trauma patient into treatment as quickly as possible. First and foremost, that involves moving the casualty to a sheltered, warm environment. *Shelter* here can be loosely defined. In the absence of a fixed structure, the protection offered by a tent or a vehicle can benefit the patient. Once they are at least minimally sheltered, patients can be infused with warmed fluids, such as a heated sterile saline, and held in insulated sleeping bags.

After trauma patients have been stabilized and treated at the local medical facility or aid station, those who are more gravely injured are likely to require evacuation to a higher echelon of care where they can receive definitive treatment. Such scenarios require careful planning to ensure adequate access to evacuation platforms based on the estimated number of patients who might require evacuation and the rate at which they can be safely moved.[9] If access to a sufficient number of movement platforms is uncertain or not possible, planners may need to expand holding capacity at the primary operating location to act as a buffer while these patients await evacuation.

Even with access to an evacuation platform, it will be important to consider the facilities to which trauma patients will be moved. Distance to the next echelon of care, holding capacity at the destination, and the time needed to move a patient will all be key factors in determining patient outcomes. Of course, evacuation operation planning must account for environmental conditions in the Arctic. For example, the linear distance between Eielson Air Force Base and the nearest community hospital in Fairbanks, Alaska, is roughly 25 miles. Transit

---

[9]   Here, critical care patients require more-specialized medical teams to accompany them during transport. In comparison, a traditional aeromedical evacuation team can handle a larger number of ambulatory patients. These distinctions are addressed in greater detail in the next section. For general planning parameters related to patient movement, see Air Force Pamphlet 10-1403, *Air Mobility Planning Factors*, Washington, D.C.: U.S. Department of the Air Force, October 24, 2018.

time by ambulance might be only 30 minutes in midsummer, but it can easily double (or more) in inhospitable winter weather. Even then, a severe trauma patient in this area will likely require aeromedical evacuation to a higher echelon of care, such as Joint Base Elmendorf-Richardson in Anchorage, roughly a 260-mile flight. Again, such movement can prove challenging in winter conditions.

Preparing for Large-Scale Patient Movement Across CONUS

At this juncture, it is helpful to review several challenges related to the movement of patients—specifically, transporting patients from an MTF at an operating location in a combat theater to a treatment facility with a broader suite of medical capabilities to provide ongoing support. Such patients will likely require medical oversight while en route to the higher-echelon treatment facility. While patients are in transit, they are often accompanied by a medical team staffed by specialists. Moving patients by air (as opposed to ship or ground ambulance) involves additional considerations to account for lower air pressure and temperature in the cabin at altitude, as well as variability in ambient sound and vibration that could affect a patient's condition and care.

An aeromedical evacuation team, consisting of a pair of flight nurses and three medical technicians, travels with patients with less severe injuries to provide medical support. Medical evacuees who require critical care are served by a critical care air transport team aboard a flying intensive care unit. The team is staffed by three specialists: an intensivist physician (such as a surgeon or critical care doctor), a critical care nurse, and a respiratory therapist. Both aeromedical evacuation and critical care air transport teams travel with supplies and equipment suited to the patient movement mission and care in the air.

As noted, in the aftermath of an adversary strike, significant numbers of casualties would require evacuation to CONUS to receive definitive medical treatment. To help allocate necessary medical support during transit, the MHS operates coordination cells, including three theater patient movement requirements centers (TPMRCs) around the globe.[10] A TPMRC receives "validated" patients from MTFs in theater, where a physician approves them for evacuation. The TPMRC safeguards the "regulated" movement of patients, ensuring that an appropriate level of care is available both en route and at the patient's receiving location.[11]

In addition to identifying how the scale of operations would grow in future conflict, the NDS highlights the likelihood of challenges to sustained freedom of movement for U.S. military assets, including aeromedical evacuation platforms. Coupled with the challenges of moving casualties at scale, patients could arrive at airfields in CONUS at irregular intervals and in large numbers. If patients also arrive by ship at seaports, this would compound the irregular timing and significant scale of arrivals. Given the constrained holding and treatment capacity at nearby CONUS MTFs, it would be challenging to accommodate all surge patients in the vicinity of these airfields and ports.

DoD has mechanisms in place to move patients to facilities with sufficient capacity and capability to treat them. Critical links in the system include managing and assigning hospital beds to incoming patients, handing off accountability for patients to the military services, tracking medical holding capacity near the locations where patients will arrive in CONUS, and allocating ground transportation assets to move patients to and from health care facilities. As the tempo of operations increases, the DoD CONUS patient reception and distribution mission must be scalable to meet growing demand.

However, the rights and authorities for regulated patient movement in CONUS were initially mapped prior to the release of the 2018 NDS. In accordance with defense planning guidelines of the time, large-scale patient movement within CONUS was envisioned more as a function of defense support to civil authorities. In this case, the predicate was not one of patient movement in the wake of a large-scale

---

[10] TPMRC East operates from Ramstein Air Base in Germany, TPMRC West is located at Joint Base Pearl Harbor–Hickam in Hawaii, and TPMRC Americas coordinates movement from Scott Air Force Base in Illinois.

[11] Michael P. Kleiman, "Global Patient Movement: Moving America's Ill and Injured Warfighters Safely, Securely, Soundly," U.S. Air Force, October 5, 2019.

conflict but, rather, patient support in the aftermath of a natural disaster or other domestic incident.[12] Under these conditions, the existing architecture of rights and authorities was more likely to be centered on civilian entities, such as the Federal Emergency Management Agency. The evolving global security picture detailed in the 2018 NDS requires reconsidering the existing rights and authorities in preparation for the large-scale movement of *combat* casualties across CONUS.

Recognizing that organic military transport assets, movement teams, and MTF beds could become more difficult to source in such a scenario, DoD could expand its patient movement options to include contracted alternatives. Similarly, patient care destinations could be augmented to include U.S. Department of Veterans Affairs treatment facilities and civilian health care networks. However, given that these options have not been implemented in real time or at scale since World War II, the authorities and data systems to regulate patient movement in this cross-agency fashion are, at best, poorly understood and infrequently exercised.

In a resource-limited environment, it can prove difficult to rapidly match a patient with an MTF with available capacity, as well as with an aircraft and the medical personnel, equipment, and supplies to support the en route care. Given that the United States has not seen a demand for large-scale casualty patient movement in several decades, neither combatant commanders nor the MHS leadership has had to grapple with real-time decisionmaking in this context. Such conditions could include the need to hold large numbers of patients at staging facilities for days at a time until aeromedical evacuation crews or patient movement assets become available.

Network conditions and capabilities could also limit the ability to rapidly and effectively execute patient reception and distribution operations. For example, limits on support for patient movement operations at certain airfields could limit patient throughput. Similarly, limits on the speed with which aeromedical evacuation crews and supplies can be

---

[12] Michael P. Kleiman, "U.S. Transportation Command Manages the Movement of America's Wounded Warfighters from Overseas to the Final Medical Treatment Destination Stateside," U.S. Air Force, January 8, 2020.

refreshed to support patient movement could bound the rate at which patients can be moved to their end destinations for definitive care. In these cases, clearer real-time SA of system constraints could improve the speed of regulated patient movement.

Overall, to better prepare for the possibility of large-scale patient reception and distribution operations in CONUS, the MHS would benefit from a fresh look at the sufficiency of the extant architecture of rights and authorities for this mission. Doing so would help the MHS identify gaps and possible mitigation strategies and mechanisms to develop an updated set of rights, authorities, systems, and supporting capabilities. In addition to exploring authorities and responsibilities, this examination could include materiel and personnel solutions. For example, staffing of aeromedical evacuation and critical care air transport teams might be inadequate to support moving patients both to and within CONUS, with shortfalls in key medical equipment, such as portable ventilators for critical care patients. Such an evaluation should highlight opportunities to improve the overall scalability and performance of CONUS patient reception and distribution.

Conclusions

This chapter examined the implications of the threat scenarios outlined in the 2018 NDS for medical support—not only on far-away battlefields but also much closer to home. Example scenarios explored how an adversary might find military installations in the Arctic circle to be convenient targets in a strike against the homeland. If U.S. forces deployed to defend the Arctic perimeter came under attack, the extreme climate would have special ramifications for combat casualty care there.

Furthermore, as casualties flowed to the homeland, whether from the Arctic or another combat theater, they could arrive in such large numbers that the current system of patient regulation would be sorely taxed in ensuring sufficient en route care resources and in allocating those patients to MTFs with available space and resources for their treatment and recovery. In planning for such scenarios, the MHS might consider new partnerships, data systems, training programs, and investments in medical equipment and materiel as means to limit potential shortfalls in the provision of casualty care.

The next chapter expands this discussion of potential shortfalls to one more element of medical materiel. Namely, the MHS effects of materiel shortfalls could ripple farther upstream in medical supply chains, where demand for consumables during large-scale combat operations could outstrip the industrial base's ability to supply them.

CHAPTER SEVEN

Improving Casualty Support Through Enhanced Resilience in Medical Supply Chains

This report has noted several challenges to treating patients in the aftermath of mass casualty events. Surges of patients stemming from large-scale missile strikes could overwhelm the treatment facilities closest to combat action. At these MTFs, demand for beds and caregiver time would quickly outstrip available patient holding capacity and the limited number of medical providers.

At this stage, a fundamental question remains: Given that the expeditionary care network might be hard pressed to meet large-scale surges of combat casualties, how might the corresponding upswell in demand for medical consumables stress production lines across the industrial base's medical supply chain? This chapter explores the ramifications for the MHS, including the conditions under which the casualty care network could run out of key lifesaving medical supplies.

Promoting Resilience in Blood Supply Chains

An important element of medical supply to support combat operations is blood. After a blast event, many of the injured will require a transfusion at some point during the course of their treatment. Blood and specialty blood products, such as plasma and red blood cells, can come from several sources. Blood can be shipped to expeditionary MTFs from collection centers in CONUS, or it can be supplied locally through on-site collection drives. Given that most blood products must be refrigerated or frozen, special handling protocols are required to ensure its safe storage. Moreover, blood loses its potency over time, and supplies must be managed with expiration dates in mind. Figure 7.1 provides an overview of the blood supply from delivery to an MTF and to its use in treating patients.

Prior analysis has shown that, under challenging CDO combat conditions, MTFs could have difficulty keeping sufficient quantities of blood and blood products on hand.[1] Although it may be possible to collect sufficient volumes of blood at donor centers across the military network, ensuring that enough is available at forward MTFs during times of need can prove challenging. The core difficulties here are twofold. First, it can be difficult to predict where demand surges will occur, especially at the outset of a conflict. Second, distribution of blood to forward MTFs can be complicated by the disruptive influence of the CDO environment, in which the adversary is able to limit the freedom of movement not only for combat forces but also for resupply vehicles.

There are several approaches that can overcome limitations in available supply. Local blood collection can help reduce the length of

Figure 7.1
Qualitative Overview of Stocks and Flows of Blood at an MTF

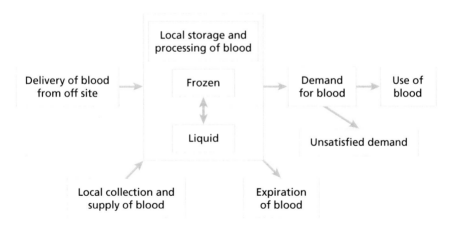

SOURCE: Thomas et al., 2018, p. 12, Figure 2.1.

---

[1]   For more on these challenges and how a portfolio approach may be required to facilitate investments in their mitigation, see Thomas et al., 2018.

the supply chain, made possible by investments in blood collection equipment, such as collection bags, needles, and sterile tubing. To help overcome challenges in the final leg of distribution to a forward MTF, autonomous drones can deliver blood and other medical supplies from medical warehouses, as discussed in Chapter Three.[2] Overall, the portfolio of mitigation strategies that the MHS invests in will ultimately depend on the nature of the conflict, in terms of the number of potential casualties, extent of the demand signals for blood, and the threat conditions under which medical support must operate.

Evaluating Resilience in the Broader Medical Supply Chain

Any discussion of potential mitigations to increase access to blood during a conflict raises a broader question: Could medical providers face similar problems sustaining on-hand stocks of other medical supplies, such as pharmaceuticals? One hypothesis is that the supply of pharmaceutical products is more robust. For example, the class of blood products is relatively narrow, and treatment protocols for combat casualties typically leave little room for substitution across a narrow array of blood products. In comparison, there is a broad industrial base for pharmaceuticals that generates a diverse array of products. If a required drug is out of stock, there is often an acceptable substitute. Additionally, drugs might be available across highly distributed production and warehousing networks, shrinking distances between product and patient.

This section uses saline, a common medical supply, to test the viability of this hypothesis and examine how its availability in the United States was affected by a natural disaster.

---

[2]   As noted in Chapter Three, Zipline, a commercial firm, is delivers blood and blood products by drone in both Ghana and Rwanda. For more on the engineering factors involved in standing up a fleet of drones for blood resupply missions, refer to Gilmore et al., 2019.

Case Study: Saline Availability in the Wake of Hurricane Maria

Saline, made by mixing sodium chloride with water, is a versatile product. Through intravenous administration, saline helps patients suffering from dehydration or dilutes a patient's medications. Applied topically, saline can be used to clean wounds. It can also be found in a variety of other products, such as eye drops and contact lens cleaning fluid. To ensure its safe use across this broad spectrum of applications, saline solutions must be produced in a specialized sterile water facility.

In the United States, saline has three main manufacturers: Baxter, ICU Medical, and Braun.[3] Of the three, Baxter is the largest producer and manufactures more than 40 percent of the total U.S. supply at its facility in Puerto Rico. Financial incentives for manufacturers have made Puerto Rico's business climate attractive to the pharmaceutical industry as a whole, and the island accounts for 10 percent of U.S. pharmaceutical production. These financial incentives help offset risk to the industry, an important consideration because the region experiences frequent tropical storms and hurricanes. On balance, the opportunities for cost savings by producing goods in Puerto Rico outweigh the risk of temporary production outages in the aftermath of a storm.

In Puerto Rico, the pharmaceutical industry, among others, stands to gain from economies of agglomeration, the geographic centralization of several major entities in a common industry. For example, multiple firms can draw on a large, trained labor pool, save costs by using common suppliers (themselves operating at larger economies of scale), and share access to well-developed energy and transportation infrastructure with the capacity to support multiple entities in the same manufacturing sector. However, when agglomerations grow overly large, they can yield significant disadvantages. In particular, when a large fraction of an industry is geographically centralized, the industry as a whole is more susceptible to disruptions from a regional natural disaster.

---

[3] ICU Medical acquired its saline production capacity from Pfizer in 2017. See ICU Medical, "Integrating ICU Medical Infusion Devices with Hospital EHR Decreased Major Dosing Errors by 52 Percent," press release, February 6, 2017.

Such a large-scale event occurred when Hurricane Maria struck Puerto Rico in September 2017. The hurricane disrupted operations at three Baxter facilities in Puerto Rico, and, to a lesser extent, facilities operated by Bristol-Myers Squibb and Pfizer. Baxter had a contingency plan in place and had invested in diesel generators to sustain power to its facilities. However, in the aftermath of Maria, diesel fuel was in short supply and high demand, compounded by a disrupted transportation and infrastructure network.[4] With its saline production facility offline for "multiple production days," Baxter reported a $70 million loss in revenue. Nevertheless, the company's third-quarter earnings in calendar year 2017 were $2.7 billion, suggesting that saline sales represent only a small fraction of its overall revenues.[5]

It is difficult to quantify the potential health consequences of disruptions to the saline supply due to Hurricane Maria. However, health care providers nationwide did note that they faced considerable challenges securing sufficient saline to meet demand during the 2017–2018 flu season.[6] To help alleviate shortages, the U.S. Food and Drug Administration (FDA) granted Baxter waivers to import saline from its overseas production facilities in Ireland and Australia to augment U.S. domestic availability.[7]

Hurricane Maria did more than temporarily disrupt saline production, with the duration of shortages compounded by a seasonal spike in demand for saline products. However, analysis is beginning to show that Maria exposed the broader struggles of an already stressed

---

[4] It is worth highlighting the parallels here between natural disaster and CDO environments. In the context of recovery from Hurricane Maria, Puerto Rico faced disruptions in the availability of key infrastructure, such as energy distribution, and degraded freedom of movement into and across the region.

[5] Eric Palmer, "Baxter Expects $70M Sales Hit from Hurricane Damage; Amgen Says Costs Could Top $165M," *Fierce Pharma*, October 15, 2017b.

[6] For example, see Peter Loftus and Jonathan D. Rockoff, "Baxter Says Saline Shipments Disrupted in Hurricane-Wracked Puerto Rico," *Wall Street Journal*, September 27, 2017, and Morten Wendelbo and Christine Crudo Blackburn, "A Saline Shortage This Flu Season Exposes a Flaw in Our Medical Supply Chain," *Smithsonian Magazine*, January 22, 2018.

[7] Zachary Brennan, "FDA Allows Temporary Saline Imports to Deal with Shortages Caused by Hurricane Maria," *Regulatory Focus*, October 11, 2017.

industry. An examination of saline shortages reported to the FDA indicated that saline lines had been stressed *continuously* since 2013, with periodic shortages reaching as far back as 2007. Industry reports to the FDA reflected not only manufacturing delays due to the hurricane but also unspecified challenges in manufacturing and the industry's ability to fully satisfy demand from the open marketplace.[8]

Given this evidence of the duration of challenges to the medical community's ability to secure a reliable saline supply, government officials suspected that the shortages might be artificial, driven by industry collusion in an effort to raise prices. Noting that Baxter and Pfizer/ICU Medical control 90 percent of the U.S. saline market, the U.S. Department of Justice initiated a federal grand jury probe in the Eastern District of Pennsylvania in 2017.[9] Over the course of the two-year investigation, the department found no compelling evidence of collusion. It ultimately closed the antitrust case and cleared each of the industry's manufacturers.[10]

These events suggest that the saline industry is indeed operating at full capacity. Given the relatively low profit margins generated from saline sales, manufacturers might have limited incentive to expand their manufacturing facilities to augment production. Coupled with a high degree of centralization, the industry is at risk of failing to meet U.S. demand for saline should production disruptions occur. Similarly, should demands spike, domestic facilities likely have limited surge capacity to meet them, forcing the FDA to consider alternative sources of supply. Saline is just one example of the potential challenges across

---

[8] Shortages crossed a number of product lines, including small- and large-volume bags of saline and saline products used for wound irrigation. Maryann Mazer-Amirshahi and Erin R. Fox, "Saline Shortages—Many Causes, No Simple Solution," *New England Journal of Medicine*, Vol. 378, No. 16, April 19, 2018.

[9] Braun is the third-largest player in this market, supplying the remainder of saline to U.S. consumers. For more, see Eric Palmer, "Pfizer Subpoenaed to Testify in DOJ's Antitrust Probe of Saline Shortages," *Fierce Pharma*, April 20, 2017, and Bowdeya Tweh, "Justice Department Investigating Baxter Over Saline Shortage," *Wall Street Journal*, May 5, 2017.

[10] Fink Densford, "Baxter Cleared from DoJ Antitrust Saline Probe," *Drug Delivery Business News*, February 1, 2019, and Nate Raymond, "U.S. Closes IV Solution Shortage Antitrust Probe, Baxter Says," Reuters, February 22, 2019.

the industrial base of medical supplies that could have implications for U.S. combat operations.

Evaluating Surge Capacity in the Pharmaceutical Industrial Base

In addition to examining challenges in saline production, it is worth exploring whether other medical consumables might see similar periodic shortages. To enhance public visibility of these issues, the FDA regularly updates a highly detailed roster of drug shortages in the United States.[11] The FDA encourages self-reporting from industrial manufacturers about the status of their product lines. It also compares market sales data against aggregated consumer requests for medical supplies. When a mismatch between supply and demand emerges, the FDA reports on the shortfall.

In their self-reports to the FDA, manufacturers are asked to assign a cause for these shortages. Most frequently, producers mark one of two categories: a known manufacturing problem that affects production or an unknown factor that has caused demand for a product to outstrip production capacity. In this latter category, it seems reasonable that a manufacturer might lack clear visibility into the root cause behind consumer demand. Similarly, a single industry producer might not have strong SA of where other producers are encountering manufacturing disruptions that contribute to a broader marketwide mismatch between supply and demand.

In terms of the scope and scale of these mismatches, the data suggest that the problem is an enduring one. Over the past two decades, an average of almost 130 drug shortages have been reported every year. Since 2014, there have been, on average, more than 200 active drug shortages in any given quarter.[12] The drugs span a range

---

[11] U.S. Food and Drug Administration, "FDA Drug Shortages: Current and Resolved Drug Shortages and Discontinuations Reported to FDA," data set, undated.

[12] American Society of Health-System Pharmacists, "Drug Shortages Statistics," webpage, undated.

of categories—from crystalloid fluids, such as saline, to chemotherapy drugs, cardiovascular medications, and antibiotics. Industry watchdogs and journalists have been increasingly focused on challenges to medication access. A common theme has emerged: Shortages are especially problematic when they affect inexpensive medications, for which the industry's profit margins are slimmest.[13]

When it comes to lines with low profit margins, a manufacturer will be drawn to opportunities to produce the good at a significant economy of scale. For example, it might operate a large production facility so it can capitalize on the cost savings of larger-scale production, including

- greater bargaining opportunity for bulk buys of raw materials
- lower shipping costs per unit, especially when full truckloads can be transported and when units can be shipped by sea freight
- training staff in larger cohorts
- maintaining a low fraction of management overhead.

A manufacturer might opt to take on higher operational costs to better capitalize on cost savings in other domains. For example, in deciding whether to move a production facility offshore, a manufacturer would expect increases in the costs of transporting goods to the United States and in delivery timelines between the production facility and U.S. customers. It might also require more warehouses in the vicinity of the production facility to house goods awaiting transport. However, the opportunity to reduce costs through a more attractive tax rate or to benefit from a more cost-effective labor pool could significantly offset these cost increases. Similarly, as noted earlier, opportunities to achieve economies of agglomeration can further support cost reductions and efficiencies in product manufacturing.

In sum, these contributions to a product's overall unit cost can be visualized in a fashion akin to that in Figure 7.2. In a canonical economy of scale, the cost per unit to produce a good drops steadily as the

---

[13] See, for example, "A Dire Scarcity of Drugs Is Worsening, in Part, Because They Are So Cheap," *The Economist*, September 14, 2019, and Roni Caryn Rabin, "Why Lifesaving Drugs May Be Missing on Your Next Flight," *New York Times*, October 3, 2019.

Figure 7.2
Idealized Economy of Scale, Including Surge Capacity

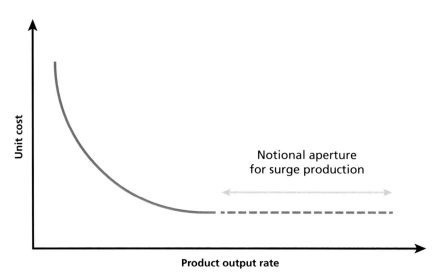

firm increases its production rate through cost-efficient investments in manufacturing equipment, labor, and facilities. Eventually, efficiencies can no longer be gained through increases in the rate of production. Ideally, the firm will opt to reserve a fraction of production capacity to meet periodic surges in demand—and to do so in a way that preserves (or only modestly increases) the cost per unit.

However, in the case of product shortages related to low-cost pharmaceuticals, it appears that, at worst, industry producers are unable to increase their production rates to meet surges in demand. At best, they may be unable to surge in a fashion that preserves the unit cost achieved at the current level of production. Under these conditions, the market could be driven into what economists term a *natural monopoly* (or oligopoly, if a few manufacturers dominate the market). Here, market conditions support a few firms operating at or near optimal scale economies. Their rates of production will likely be able to satisfy steady-state demands, but shortages might arise during periods of greater-than-expected demand. Given the cost of entry for a new firm to enter the market, as well as the slender profit margins available to aid that firm in recapturing its investment cost, additional competition is discouraged.

These conditions also suggest that, should increased production rates be possible, manufacturers might operate at a significant diseconomy of scale, as shown in Figure 7.3. Given that U.S. firms have not scaled up production during historical periods of surge demand for many low-cost drugs, these producers might face steep cost disincentives to do so. For example, their suppliers may not be able to offer the necessary raw materials at scale or to do so without significantly increasing their own unit costs. Similarly, to scale up production, the firm might identify a need for additional infrastructure—for example, to support increases in energy, storage, and transportation—to produce and distribute goods. Access to energy can be particularly limiting; a production facility's local power grid might be unable to support the manufacturer's request for an increase in supply. Similarly, access to skilled labor can become a limiting factor if additional shifts cannot be staffed, if there is a shortage of workers to operate highly specialized machinery, or if this machinery is already operating at capacity.

Figure 7.3
Canonical Diseconomy of Scale

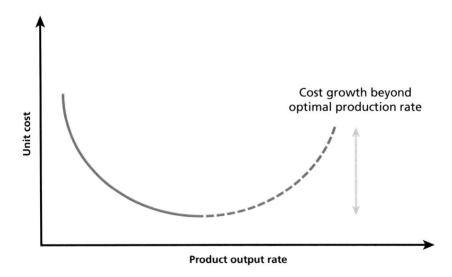

The Challenge of Counterfeit Drugs in the Global Supply

It is worth noting that the regulatory environment for drug manufacturing in the United States is strong. A precondition for pharmaceutical manufacturers to operate or do business in the United States is that, with FDA oversight, drugs will be produced under high quality-control standards. In other nations, including India and China, industry regulations are not as strong as in the United States. As a consequence, manufacturers in these overseas markets might find profitable opportunities to fill niche demands for low-cost drugs—say, in the production of generic antibiotics. To successfully compete in a cost-competitive marketplace, producers might locate their manufacturing and distribution in a region with less restrictive regulatory oversight where they can enjoy a lower investment in quality assurance and control. Consequently, these products can suffer from defects, such as contamination or degraded potency, that are less common in well-regulated markets. Some of these manufacturers might produce drugs for which they are unlicensed or uncertified, thereby defrauding the entity that holds the legal rights to their manufacture. For the purposes of this discussion, *counterfeit* is used as an umbrella term referring to the combined classes of subpotent, degraded, and illegally produced drugs.[14]

Counterfeits have filled the gap between limited access to regulated drugs and their vastly larger global demand. The challenge of counterfeits entering the market has been especially problematic in Africa and Asia. Across these regions, awareness of the problem among political leadership is sometimes limited, including both the public health and economic ramifications. Furthermore, governments can be constrained in their ability to enforce regulations by the manpower available to staff inspection teams, limited authority to access and inspect laboratories and testing equipment, or a limited pool of labor to operate technologically advanced testing systems.[15]

---

[14] From a stricter legal vantage, *counterfeit* refers specifically to drugs produced with an intent to deceive consumers or to defraud licensed manufacturers.

[15] Muhammad H. Zaman, *Bitter Pills: The Global War on Counterfeit Drugs*, New York: Oxford University Press, 2018.

Although the centers of gravity for counterfeit drugs are in Asia and Africa, the problem is by no means restricted to those regions. Occasionally, these materials are discovered in the U.S. pharmaceutical industrial base. For example, one serious incident occurred when contaminated precursors used in the anticoagulant drug heparin made their way from a production facility in China into the U.S. manufacturing base. In 2008, the heparin produced with this contaminated ingredient was distributed to U.S. hospitals, killing more than 80 patients and injuring almost 800 more. The FDA had developed a testing protocol for the contamination, but it lacked the authority to mandate testing. Furthermore, in the absence of U.S. supplies of the ingredient, the FDA allowed drug companies to import of the heparin precursor from China because it feared a shortage of the drug.[16]

It is important to note that the technologies available for detecting counterfeits are limited, and these tests are sensitive to context. For example, depending on whether an inspector is looking for a specific contaminant or assessing the amount of a drug's active ingredient, the necessary testing equipment, methods, and reagents will vary. There are important ramifications for the MHS because it is difficult to develop, *a priori*, a one-size-fits-all kit for deploying testing capabilities to a combat zone. However, a range of promising technologies has begun to emerge, from using a smartphone to identify counterfeits based on a pill's configuration to testing for the concentration of active ingredients using paper strips and employing portable microfluidic technologies for rapid drug assays.[17]

---

[16] Waivers of this nature are not unusual, especially for drugs and drug precursors that are made largely overseas. At the time, China produced half of the world supply of heparin's active pharmaceutical ingredient. For more, see U.S. House of Representatives, Committee on Energy and Commerce, Subcommittee on Oversight and Investigation, "The Heparin Disaster: Chinese Counterfeits and American Failures," hearing transcript, Washington, D.C., April 29, 2008.

[17] Yepoka Yeebo, "The African Startup Using Phones to Spot Counterfeit Drugs," *Bloomberg Businessweek*, July 31, 2015; Kirsty Oswald, "US$1 Test Card Can Detect Poor Quality Ceftriaxone Antibiotic," *Pharmaceutical Journal*, August 31, 2016; George M. Whitesides, "The Origins and the Future of Microfluidics," *Nature*, Vol. 442, No. 7107, July 27, 2006.

In terms of broader measures to secure the medical supply chain, partner nations might need better options to detect and remove counterfeits.[18] As noted earlier, a partner might have limited access to a sufficiently trained technological workforce to operate testing equipment. Furthermore, once the procurement, operational, and sustainment costs for running the equipment are tallied, it is important to ensure that the partner can support the cost per test so that testing for counterfeits remains an enduring capability. It is also worth highlighting that, to be conducted at scale, testing has to be both cost-effective and fast enough to meet demand. In concert, these capabilities can boost supply chain resilience and enhance drug safety worldwide.

Incentivizing Flexibility in the Medical Supply Industrial Base

So far, this chapter has addressed several domains related to ensuring resilience in medical supply chains. Solutions ranged from ensuring access to supplies to meet surge demand, especially for pharmaceuticals and other consumables, to increasing confidence that counterfeits have not crept into available supplies. At the heart of this discussion were mechanisms for reducing the risk of harm to deployed forces by ensuring access to safe medical supplies in times of need to treat casualties.

Framing Risk in the Context of Access to Medical Materiel

DoD and industry agree on the principal drivers of risk in the medical supply chain. Namely, they see risk as a failure to satisfy one of four conditions: the required quantity of a good, the schedule for supplying that good, its price, and its quality.[19] This is especially true in the steady-state environment, in which both supplier and buyer seek to

---

[18] Stephanie Kovacs, Stephen E. Hawes, Stephen N. Maley, Emily Mosites, Ling Wong, and Andy Stergachis, "Technologies for Detecting Falsified and Substandard Drugs in Low and Middle-Income Countries," *PLoS One*, Vol. 9, No. 3, March 26, 2014.

[19] This basic framing of risk stems from International Risk Governance Center, *Introduction to the IRGC Risk Governance Framework*, rev. ed., Lausanne, Switzerland, 2017.

uphold arrangements facilitating access to the right product and surety of its safety and efficacy, shipped at the right time, and at the agreed-upon price.

In the context of large-scale contingency support, these parties' risk metrics might diverge. Industry partners will likely continue to frame risk mitigation as the driver to limit the extent of *unmet contractual obligation*. This is a common metric in evaluating the performance of product supply chains. However, DoD will likely begin to view risk management as an effort to limit the extent of *unmet demands across the network of care*. Here, with an eye toward ensuring product quality, DoD might wish to expand the quantity of available goods at an accelerated schedule, and the initially agreed-upon price for those goods might no longer be a binding constraint. Appreciating these two different approaches to risk is key to evaluating where there might be opportunities to ensure access to medical supplies in times of urgent need.

Mitigating Risk Through Flexibility

Supply chain entities can help manage risk by preparing to exercise a degree of flexibility in their manufacturing processes. One useful definition of *flexibility* is "the ability to respond to change without increasing operational and supply chain costs and with little or no delay in response time."[20] This definition of *flexibility* can apply to three key domains: system, process, and product. In process flexibility, a firm employs mechanisms to mitigate excessive wait times in the manufacturing process, such as load-balancing production equipment and improving staff utilization by cross-training them in key skills.[21] In product flexibility, a firm develops a modular product architecture or makes more-substitutable products. Here, the manufacturer can

---

[20] David M. Upton, "The Management of Manufacturing Flexibility," *California Management Review*, Vol. 36, No. 2, 1994.

[21] Seyed M. R. Irvani, "Design and Control Principles of Flexible Workforce in Manufacturing Systems" in James J. Cochran, Louis A. Cox, Jr., Pinar Keskinocak, Jeffrey P. Kharoufeh, and J. Cole Smith, eds., *Wiley Encyclopedia of Operations Research and Management Science*, Hoboken, N.J.: Wiley, 2011.

more readily flex to respond to changes in the mix or size of customer orders.[22]

Given the specificity of product requirements in the medical supply industry—especially in pharmaceuticals—system flexibility can offer manufacturers the greatest opportunity to manage risk. Here, flexibility is achieved through mechanisms to improve SA of inventory levels, backlogs, and the availability of production equipment. System flexibility can also be achieved through investments that allow manufacturing facilities to produce multiple products. With these capabilities, the manufacturer will be poised to more readily identify changing demand patterns, both geographically and over time. As these evolving demand trends are detected, the network of production facilities can adapt to cost-effectively satisfy global customer demands. Although there is a need to invest in these capabilities, analysis has shown that these costs can be recovered through reductions in operational costs, reductions in order response time, and improved service levels.[23]

Flexibility is also an important consideration in the context of MHS operations. The MHS not only needs to support day-to-day care in garrison, but it also needs to prepare to provide medical support in combat scenarios. There are two general areas in which the MHS can enhance its flexibility: uncertainty in pending demands for medical supplies and expected lead times to receive orders. This tradespace is depicted in Figure 7.4.

In the steady-state environment, in which SA of on-hand stock levels is high and orders from suppliers are expected to arrive quickly, the MHS can operate in a mode of continuous replenishment for many common consumables, routinely restocking such goods as bandages and saline. Because demand for some niche products may be more uncertain, such as for specialty blood products, these orders can be placed on an as-needed basis. This practice was also referred to as "pull" logistics in Chapter Five.

---

[22] Jayashankar M. Swaminathan, "Enabling Customization Using Standardized Operations," *California Management Review*, Vol. 43, No. 3, Spring 2001.

[23] David Simchi-Levi, *Operations Rules: Delivering Customer Value Through Flexible Operations*, Cambridge, Mass.: MIT Press, 2010.

Figure 7.4
Operational Strategies Based on Lead Time and Demand Uncertainty

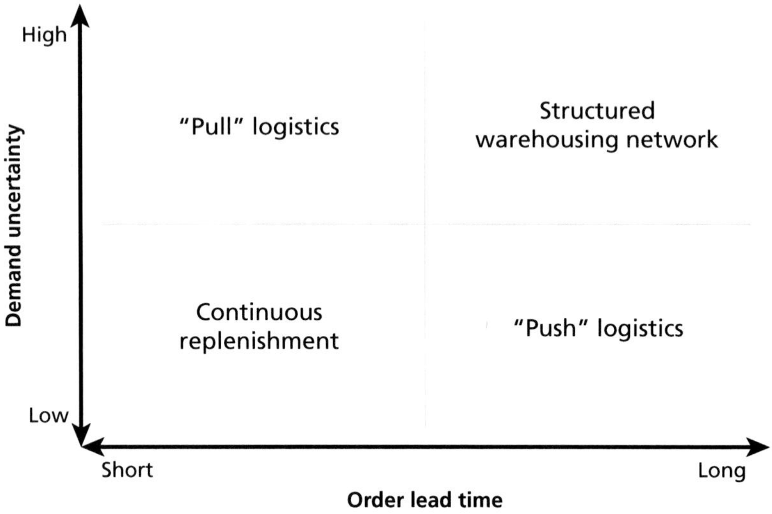

SOURCE: Adapted from Simchi-Levi, 2010, p. 45, Figure 3.3. Used with permission.

However, order lead times can grow considerably during combat operations, especially for resupply orders that must be shipped from CONUS to overseas contingency locations. When demand uncertainty is low, such as when casualties are expected at larger operating locations, data systems might not require a continuous uplink. Even in the absence of a request for supplies, it can prove beneficial to route "push" logistics packages of commonly used trauma supplies to those locations, such as units of saline and packed red blood cells. Finally, in combat environments, a globally distributed medical WRM network can help expedite requests to meet unexpected demands for specialty equipment and supplies, such as portable heart monitors and ventilators for patients requiring evacuation.

It is worth highlighting that strategies can change as conditions evolve. Consider, for example, how communication links tend to be more reliable later in a conflict as U.S. forces are able to drive an adversary from the battlefield. Similarly, the medical enterprise would have more-dependable SA of goods on the shelves at forward MTFs. Consequently, sustainment strategies at that these sites could advance from receiving "push" packages of a predetermined configuration to a state of continuous and highly tailored replenishment based on their individual needs.

Incentivizing Flexibility Among MHS Suppliers

As noted earlier, a wide array of low-cost medical supplies populate the FDA's roster of goods in shortage, including generic pharmaceuticals. Given that these goods have a low profit margin, there will likely be little incentive for the industrial base to change its practices. For example, with limited, if any, financial gains to be realized by expanding production rates, manufacturers have limited motive to invest in building surge capacity for key drug lines.

It may be necessary to explore whole-of-government approaches to motivate change and promote supply chain resilience. For example, there are clear and common ties in the need for resilient access to medical supplies in both combat support and disaster response. Consequently, several government entities could spearhead programs to incentivize such activities, including the Office of the Under Secretary of Defense for Acquisition and Sustainment, the FDA, and the U.S. Department of State.

Through a coalition approach, flexibility in the industrial base could be achieved by prioritizing access to medical supplies in support of both national defense and public health. For example, federal officials could target investments toward international manufacturers to help them improve their production and quality assurance processes to meet FDA standards for drugs and medical equipment. This would act as a mechanism to both diversify and expand the industrial base. Investments could also target projects to enhance utility and transportation infrastructure in regions where industrial development is constrained by shortages of these resources. Additionally, to shorten medical supply chains and to increase their security and oversight, U.S. firms could receive financial incentives to "redomicile" the production of key drugs and their active ingredients in the United States. France recently launched such an initiative as a means to increase domestic drug security, and the United States has taken initial steps to do so under the Defense Production Act in light of challenges during the global coronavirus pandemic.[24]

Linking Resilient Medical Supply Chains to Combat Outcomes

Rounding out the discussion in this chapter is a case study of a hypothetical scenario. Here, a fictional future combat operation illustrates the possible ramifications of relying on a potentially fragile pharmaceutical industrial base. Given the scenarios posited by the 2018 NDS, it is important to consider how medical supply chains could be stressed under the conditions of large-scale combat. As noted, even during peacetime, these issues can be relevant, such as when the MHS is called upon to support large-scale HADR operations.

Case Study: A Vignette of Medical Support in a Hypothetical High-End Fight

In 2030, the United States enters a large-scale conflict with peer adversary in support of the national defense of its long-term strategic partners and allies. At the outset of the conflict, to limit freedom of movement for U.S. forces, adversary forces levy protracted missile strikes at U.S. operating locations across the theater. However, given the vast number of missiles employed, U.S. defenses barely diminish the volume of most of the adversary's salvos. The missiles that successfully breach the defense network yield tens of thousands of casualties over the first few weeks of the war. As casualties flood expeditionary MTFs, thousands need to be treated for serious blast injuries, such as burns, shrapnel wounds, and broken limbs.

Given the severity and geographic extent of these strikes, U.S. partners across the region fear attacks against their own critical infra-

---

[24] "A Dire Scarcity of Drugs Is Worsening, in Part, Because They Are So Cheap," 2019; J. Edward Moreno, "Kodak Wins $765M Federal Loan in Push to Produce Domestic Pharmaceuticals," *The Hill*, July 28, 2020.

structure, possibly leading to large-scale civilian casualties. Consequently, partner-nation hospitals deny admission to wounded U.S. personnel, reserving bed space for their own expected casualties. With a lack of higher-echelon care available to treat the most seriously injured U.S. troops, these casualties must be evacuated back to CONUS for their definitive medical treatment.

However, many of the adversary's missiles have targeted air bases, damaging such key infrastructure as runways and fuel reserves. In this contested environment, casualties can be evacuated only during brief windows of opportunity. Thus, forward MTFs must hold more trauma patients than their planned capacity, and they must hold them longer than in any conflict in the past century.

To provide care to these large numbers of casualties in the combat theater, commanders quickly recognize that it is essential to conserve medical supplies. Degraded freedom of movement limits not only the generation of combat power but also the agile resupply of key sustainment lines, including medical materiel. Given resource drawdowns in recent decades to support a robust medical WRM posture, reserves in these strategic stockpiles have dwindled. With constrained options for rapid resupply, spikes in the demand for medical supplies frequently exhaust on-hand stocks at deployed MTFs. Moreover, access to generic drugs, such as antibiotics, is especially limited.

Drawing on small quantities of on-hand stock, MTFs rapidly run out of supplies to ward off infection, driving supply officers to scour local markets for antibiotics. Not only are local supplies scant but, commingled with the pharmaceutical-grade legal drugs, there is a significant volume of counterfeit medications. Antibiotic therapy with the wrong drugs, potency, or duration allows invading microbial strains to evolve resistance to future treatment. Consequently, the rate and severity of infection among trauma patients rises rapidly across the network of expeditionary MTFs. Even when FDA-approved supplies arrive in medical resupply packages from CONUS, infections stemming from these new antimicrobial-resistant (AMR) pathogens prove stubbornly resistant to treatment.[25]

Under less strenuous combat conditions, many of the wounded could have been treated for their light burns and shrapnel injuries and returned to their duty stations. However, with the pervasive and growing level of AMR infection among those with otherwise non–life-threatening wounds, many troops are unable to readily return to their combat stations. With this restricted ability to rapidly reconstitute the force, understaffing among frontline combat units drives the United States to remain in operations designed to blunt the adversary's advance for a protracted period, allowing enemy forces a significant combat advantage in the initial stages of the war.

As combat conditions permit, waves of patients now infected with AMR pathogens are evacuated to CONUS. However, the sheer volume of patients returning to these military air hubs overwhelms the availability of aircraft and medical support teams to transload them onto aircraft bound for treatment facilities closer to their home stations. As a result, patients are assigned to any hospitals with capacity to take them and where the limited number of available transport teams and assets can carry them.

To minimize wait times at air hubs, patients are evacuated to the largest U.S. cities, where hospital capacity in 2030 is more highly concentrated. Across the nationwide network, patients now contaminate crowded hospitals with AMR pathogens. Medical providers are unable to fully contain these pathogens, and AMR infection begins to spread into the largest and densest metropolitan areas.[26] Given the heavy frequency of transport between these locations and other megacities

———————————

[25] Given the limited profits in antibiotic production, industry incentives to invest in research and development for next-generation antibiotics are effectively nonexistent. Consequently, there has been less of a coordinated effort to develop new drugs in academic labs, where advances are slow, and industry faces negligible exposure to risk by investing heavily in the research and development pipeline. John LaMattina, "Universities Stepping Up Efforts to Discover Drugs," *Forbes*, October 21, 2013.

[26] Medical providers themselves can prove to be a significant vector for spreading AMR into the community. See Maryn McKenna, *Superbug: The Fatal Menace of MRSA*, New York: Free Press, 2010.

around the world, the contagion threatens the field of medicine with an imminent return to the pre-antibiotic age of World War I—and on a global stage.

As AMR contagion spreads most rapidly across the United States, confidence in health care institutions rapidly erodes. The public widely views hospitals as reservoirs of untreatable infection. Public support for DoD also rapidly wanes, given its inability to adequately treat the combat casualties that sparked the pandemic. Both Congress and the public assert that the pharmaceutical industry has failed to meet the vital interests of both public health and national security. Having conducted blunt-phase combat operations for too long with no meaningful advances against the adversary, and with political leadership facing growing pressure to stem the spread of AMR at home, the United States is compelled to prioritize the health of its citizenry over its long-standing commitments to its allies. It withdraws from the conflict, ceding to the adversary and, in the process, undermining international confidence in its ability to uphold the rule of law and to support the security of its partners.

Conclusions

This chapter examined the resilience of the U.S. industrial base for medical supplies, with a particular focus on the pharmaceutical sector. Under typical day-to-day conditions, the industry is largely capable of providing safe and effective drugs and supplies to the U.S. health care system. However, the industry has also faced significant pressure to manage costs; this has, in turn, posed challenges to the manufacture of low-cost drugs, especially in the generic pharmaceutical space. Firms have taken some steps to overcome these challenges, such as working with international partners whose production costs are lower and tailoring production capacity carefully to match expected demands.

However, with a limited ability to surge production as demands arise, many pharmaceuticals are periodically in short supply. The 2018 NDS highlights scenarios that could further stress the industrial base, creating even greater demand spikes to support casualties in a large-scale contingency. Under these surge conditions, medical providers could face significant difficulty securing sufficient quantities of key drugs.

Consequently, this chapter explored a range of mitigation strategies that the MHS could pursue in collaboration with industry and other government partners. Here, resources could be targeted toward incentivizing industry investments in surge production capacity, diversifying the industrial base, and supporting international partners in enhancing their quality assurance and quality control processes to better align with FDA practices and regulations. In so doing, the MHS can help mitigate the risk of supply shortages and promote flexibility in industrial supply chain operations.

CHAPTER EIGHT

Recommendations and Policy Implications

This report presented a wide range of challenges stemming from the evolution of the threat environment outlined in the 2018 NDS. Although the current MHS posture of combat care offers many benefits to the casualty population, potential shifts in and enhancements to that medical posture may be warranted to improve both patient and operational outcomes on a future battlefield. The mitigations explored and discussed here span a broad spectrum, including augmented training, facility tailoring, enhancements to medical logistics, and adaptations of clinical approaches, each offering the potential to improve combat casualty care in a high-intensity conventional conflict:

- *Prepare combat casualty care for a rapidly evolving set of global threats.* Rather than organizing, training, and equipping the medical force for a fight that resembles recent military operations in the Middle East, the MHS should consider how evolving threat conditions might change the requirements for medical support in a future fight. For example, adversaries are heavily investing in advanced missile systems, a combat capability that stands to generate more trauma casualties than U.S. forces have encountered in a century.
- *Forecast requirements for care on the future battlefield.* By evaluating the casualty distributions likely to be encountered in the aftermath of large-scale blast events, the MHS can better prepare to treat those injuries—and to treat them in significant numbers.
- *Enhance treatment options at and near the POI.* For example, enhancing first responders' skills can improve overall medi-

cal capability, while expanding the treatment space at field hospitals—especially in intensive care wards—can meaningfully improve medical capacity. Moreover, approaches to expedite patient throughput are equally important in improving outcomes, such as employing triage strategies specific to mass trauma events. These approaches can not only improve return to duty rates to expedite the reconstitution of the force under attack, but they can improve the odds of survival for patients with more serious combat wounds.

- *Evaluate the benefits of an expanded posture for prepositioned medical assets.* In ensuring that medical capability will be available at forward operating locations prior to the onset of hostilities, it might be important to consider approaches that were more prevalent during the Cold War era. Expanding the global network of warehouses storing medical materiel can ensure that prepositioned supplies and expeditionary facilities are immediately accessible in key threat regions.
- *Consider options to improve the resilience of medical logistics and sustainment capabilities.* Many types of medical materiel have special storage, handling, and maintenance requirements, such as a need for periodic inspection, repair, and replacement. The MHS has a number of manpower options to support these operations, but it must carefully balance the cost-saving potential of civilian and contract labor against requirements to deploy military personnel in these roles who are able provide broader support for contingency operations. Where there are gaps in asset maintenance and sustainment support, the MHS could benefit from expanded agreements with partner nations. Moreover, all medical logistics support is predicated on reliable and enduring SA of what assets are where, at what levels, and in what condition. To sustain that awareness in a contested environment during combat, the MHS might need to consider ways to enhance the resilience of key data systems and communication links.
- *Prepare for homeland support and homeland defense missions.* The 2018 NDS emphasizes not only the growing potential for conflict overseas but also the heightened need for military support closer

to home. Thus, the MHS should consider how adversary threats may drive the need for medical support in the Arctic, for example, and the ramifications for the care of trauma patients in that environment. Because large numbers of casualties could return to CONUS, the MHS would benefit from a clearer map of the rights and authorities involved in managing the flow of patients both within the MHS network and to civilian care facilities.

- *Build resilience into the industrial base for medical supplies.* In their day-to-day support to the MHS, manufacturers can generally meet contracted demands for medical supplies. However, given how the industrial base has achieved significant cost-effectiveness through advances in production efficiencies, access to some supplies could be far more constrained under the surge-demand conditions of a large-scale contingency. This may prove especially true for low-cost goods, such as saline and generic pharmaceuticals, for which supply chains can be long and the industrial base may lack meaningful surge production capacity. The MHS should consider options to diversify its partnerships with the industrial base—possibly in concert with interagency partners—and invest in enhanced manufacturing practices to more quickly meet surge-demand signals.

As discussed earlier, each of these mitigations can have significant value in improving casualty care. However, no single solution appears to be a "silver bullet" that will improve all outcomes. Thus, it is important for the MHS to develop portfolios of options and to assess each portfolio with respect to its overall cost and performance. For example, which mitigation portfolios would be most cost-effective in improving return-to-duty rates? Do they combine materiel and training solutions, such as investing in a broader network of medical WRM storage sites and expanding training for first responders? Or do they involve a shift in current policy, with increased investment in partner-nation medical support capabilities and enhancements to the industrial base for medical supplies? As the MHS evaluates these considerations, it will be better positioned to inform decisionmakers and stakeholders of key cost points and where forecasted capabilities will offer maximum benefit.

Although this report explored an array of initiatives that the MHS could consider or pursue, the discussion has only begun when it comes to MHS preparations for the evolving global threat environment. Other key domains for the MHS to investigate relate to the topics addressed in this report. The following are just a few examples:

- *Different threats.* This report focused largely on conventional missiles and blast injuries, but the NDS identifies other types of threats. For example, chemical and biological attacks require a significantly different medical response from a conventional blast, and extreme precautions must be taken to prevent contamination from spreading. A nuclear or radiological attack would also drive different response approaches and could yield significantly more casualties than the conventional attacks discussed here.
- *Austere environments.* This report addressed a range of geographic regions identified by the 2018 NDS, such as the Middle East, Europe, the Indo-Pacific, and the Arctic, as well as concerns related to large-scale casualty support. However, it did not explore the special challenges and care requirements associated with dispersed forces operating in far more austere regions, such as sub-Saharan Africa. Here, the distance between injured personnel and medical facilities can be vast, and the complexity of securing transportation and expediting patient evacuation to an appropriate MTF involves very different considerations from those for large-scale combat support in a less austere theater.[1]
- *Additional clinical interventions.* This report highlighted several potentially useful enhancements to combat casualty care, such as additional training for first responders and explicit return-to-duty protocols for patients suffering from concussions. However,

---

[1] For severely injured trauma patients, shrinking the time between injury and the patient's initial surgical interventions is especially important. See Christopher A. Mouton, Edward W. Chan, Adam R. Grissom, John P. Godges, Badreddine Ahtchi, and Brian Dougherty, *Personnel Recovery in the AFRICOM Area of Responsibility: Cost-Effective Options for Improvement*, Santa Monica, Calif.: RAND Corporation, RR-2161/1-AFRICOM, 2019.

a range of other considerations also warrant further exploration. For example, pain management can prove challenging across large populations of trauma patients. Further assessment could inform novel strategies to evaluate and treat these patients while reducing the potential for opioid addiction. Similarly, caring for patients suffering from severe burns can be resource-intensive, and supplies can be especially limited at smaller deployed MTFs. Expanding investment in burn therapies targeted toward these resource-scarce environments could significantly advance the quality of combat casualty care.

In conclusion, the 2018 NDS projects a future threat environment that is starkly different from the U.S. military's experiences in recent contingencies. This has significantly changed the operational view for front-line combat units and the capabilities they need to prepare to employ against a future adversary. To sustain the warfighter's combat capability, the combat service support functions, such as medical, are facing an equally daunting paradigm shift. Careful reflection on the challenges outlined in the 2018 NDS reveals a range of opportunities to improve the capability of the MHS in a future fight. With the objective of building a more agile force, the MHS has numerous options to bring resilient logistics and robust sustainment to its enhanced mission sets and to optimize its support for the warfighter both at home and in combat.

An Overview of Triage Principles

This report highlighted some promising strategies to improve patient outcomes in a high-intensity conventional conflict. Two key options focused on triage scenarios: (1) identifying mTBI patients and separating them from the general patient population to clear congestion at MTFs and (2) prioritizing patients for treatment differently in the event of mass trauma surges to best utilize available medical resources. Given that emphasis on triage in the suite of mitigations, it is helpful to more fully contextualize these approaches and how triage protocols are executed. To that end, this appendix presents a brief history of triage, an overview of core triage principles, and a summary of various triage strategies.

Historical Origins of Triage

Triage is derived from the French word *trier*, which means "to sort." The term refers to the allocation of scarce medical resources relative to the overall treatment needs of the patient population. There are generally three conditions that need to be met for this allocation process to be considered triage:[1]

- There is a scarcity of health care resources relative to the overall patient demand signal.

---

[1] Kenneth V. Iserson and John C. Moskop, "Triage in Medicine, Part I: Concept, History, and Types," *Annals of Emergency Medicine*, Vol. 49, No. 3, March 2007.

- A triage officer acts as a focal point to assess each patient's medical needs.
- The triage officer uses an established system or set of criteria to determine the treatment plan and priority for each patient.

Baron Dominique Jean Larrey is generally credited with establishing triage principles during the Napoleonic Wars. Trained as a surgeon in the French Army, Larrey believed that rapid medical care was the key to saving more lives. To that end, he established field hospitals as close to the battlefield as possible and prioritized patients' treatment based on the severity of their wounds. Importantly, he did not prioritize patients by nonmedical criteria, such as rank. Patients who were not in immediate danger from their wounds were sent to treatment facilities away from the battlefield, which allowed the immediate treatment of more-serious injuries. This protocol greatly reduced the mortality rate among the wounded.[2] Larrey's framework subsequently informed modern traumatology and the military systems of prehospital care based on triage and patient transport.

By World War I, the use of prehospital medical care systems on the battlefield was well established. However, since the inception of triage in the early 1800s, larger and deadlier weapons had been developed, resulting in a dramatic increase in the number of casualties on the battlefield and the severity of their wounds. As a result, triage took on a new tactical role as conserving medical manpower was prioritized over immediately treating the sick and wounded. Specifically, soldiers with minor injuries that might not hinder their effectiveness in battle were treated first and sent back into combat. This approach, oriented toward the rapid reconstitution of the force through medical care, continued during World War II.

By 1958, triage categories had evolved further. The NATO military handbook of that era described three triage categories:[3]

---

[2] Mariusz Goniewicz, "Effect of Military Conflicts on the Formation of Emergency Medical Services Systems Worldwide," *Academic Emergency Medicine*, Vol. 20, No. 5, May 2013.

[3] Iserson and Moskop, 2007.

- those with minor injuries who can return to service with treatment
- those who are seriously injured and need immediate medical care
- those who are gravely wounded and unlikely to survive, even with medical intervention.

Attention also turned to minimizing the time between injury and receipt of medical care. Medical personnel discovered that if care could be rendered within the first 60 minutes after an injury, mortality rates could be reduced. With the advent of helicopters, tactical casualty evacuation became more commonly available during the Korean and Vietnam Wars, and reducing wait times for life-saving care to within one hour was increasingly possible. This window of opportunity has become known as the "golden hour." Modern military medicine continues to explore innovative tactics, techniques, and procedures to expedite treatment and provide advanced medical care as quickly as possible.[4]

Fundamental Principles of Triage

As suggested earlier, the need for triage occurs "when the needs or demands for medical treatment significantly outstrip the available resources."[5] How these scarce resources will be distributed can be a matter of life or death to a patient, and the inputs to the decisionmaking process can provoke philosophical and ethical debate. An understanding of the underlying principles and logic behind triage strategies can help contextualize triage decisions and thereby improve how a triage officer makes these challenging choices. Figure A.1 summarizes factors that must be considered when implementing triage strategies.

The main goal of combat medicine is to "return the greatest possible number of warfighters to combat and the preservation of life, limb,

---

[4] Goniewicz, 2013.

[5] Iserson and Moskop, 2007, p. 275.

Figure A.1
Challenges to Triage Decisions

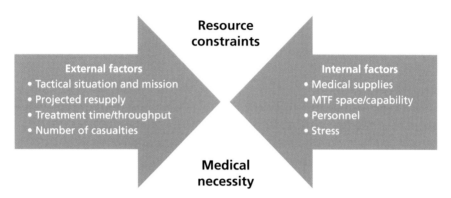

Resource
constraints

External factors
- Tactical situation and mission
- Projected resupply
- Treatment time/throughput
- Number of casualties

Internal factors
- Medical supplies
- MTF space/capability
- Personnel
- Stress

Medical
necessity

and eyesight."[6] Priority for committing resources is assigned first on the basis of the mission at hand and the underlying and prevailing tactical situation, then on the basis of a patient's injuries. Other underlying principles for distributing resources and care include the following: [7]

1. *The principle of utility.* Utilitarians believe that actions should be judged on their consequences and on the overall net benefit to the greater group. This strategy is the overarching principle that guides the U.S. military during combat operations with constrained resources. If a triage decision leads to an adverse patient outcome, a utilitarian framing could still justify that decision if the benefit to the overall patient population is greater. In practice, this principle can be difficult to put into practice—say, if a severely ill patient is left untreated so medical personnel can focus on a greater number of less severely injured patients.

2. *The difference principle.* This principle argues that medical benefits should first be distributed to those who are most in need. This approach adopts a so-called "maximin" prioritization strat-

---

[6]   U.S. Army Office of the Surgeon General, *Emergency War Surgery*, 5th rev. ed., Fort Sam Houston, Tex., 2018, p. 24.

[7]   John C. Moskop and Kenneth V. Iserson, "Triage in Medicine, Part II: Underlying Values and Principles," *Annals of Emergency Medicine*, Vol. 49, No. 3, March 2007.

egy, in which decisions are made to maximize the odds of survival for those in the population deemed "worst off." In practice during medical triage, however, it can be difficult to determine which patients are worst off. Furthermore, if severely injured patients represent a disproportionate share of casualties, it can be challenging to assess the likelihood that triage under the difference principle would yield an increase in the total number of patients who succumb to their wounds.[8]

3. *The principle of equal chances.* Advocates of the equal chances principle argue that the notion of weighing the expected value of medical intervention is inappropriate in the context of saving human lives. Instead, all patients should be afforded an equal chance of survival. In practice, this could mean treating patients on a first-come, first-served basis. In a scenario with adequate resources, this principle might be a triage officer's natural default, especially because a physician would likely struggle with the notion of turning away a patient in need of care. However, in a mass trauma scenario, an equal chances approach could lead to an overall increase in mortality across the patient population, with limited resources potentially allocated to the most gravely wounded, whose likelihood of survival is limited even with immediate medical intervention.

To help frame these triage principles in the context of combat, consider a small MTF with an on-hand supply of only 20 units of red blood cells. Assume that ten combat casualties arrive simultaneously for treatment. One is gravely wounded by a blast casualty with low odds of survival even with surgery, and who require at least 20 units of blood if admitted to the operating theater. The other nine casualties are suffering from moderate but treatable shrapnel wounds; they will be able to survive their injuries if they each receive two units of blood during treatment.

---

[8]   The difference principle here was first outlined in the context of societal benefits. See John Rawls, *A Theory of Justice*, Cambridge, Mass.: Harvard University Press, 1971.

- Utilitarian triage would likely direct palliative care to the blast victim who would most likely succumb to the wounds even with surgical intervention. The scarce blood supply would be used to treat the remaining patients.
- Triage decisions based on the difference principle would be difficult, given that all these patients may die of their wounds without treatment. However, the "worst-off" patient would be the blast casualty in urgent need of surgery; the shrapnel casualties may be able to survive until an alternative blood supply can be secured. This patient prioritization risks losing the lives of all ten patients: The blast casualty may not survive surgery, and the shrapnel casualties may not survive until blood supplies are located.
- Triage decisions based on an equal chances principle would likely prioritize treatment for the blast victim, especially if the exigency of treatment leads to the patient's admission to the MTF in advance of the other casualties. As with a decision made on the basis of the difference principle, there is a risk that all ten casualties will succumb to their wounds.

It is worth noting that life-saving triage also occurs outside the context of a mass casualty event, where the availability of time might allow an evaluation of other considerations. For example, in the scenario of allocating organs for transplantation, a range of situational factors could influence the prioritization decision, including assessing the broader societal value of the transplant patient and the potential to maximize the patient's lifespan. These considerations effectively evaluate how the care will be "used." However, in the context of the rapid decisionmaking process called for during a mass casualty event, time is of the essence, and there might be little opportunity for nuanced reflection.[9]

In sum, several considerations will come into play when making patient-prioritization decisions. In the deployed environment, military

---

[9] Douglas B. White, Mitchell H. Katz, John M. Luce, and Bernard Lo, "Who Should Receive Life Support During a Public Health Emergency? Using Ethical Principles to Improve Allocation Decisions," *Annals of Internal Medicine*, Vol. 150, No. 2, January 20, 2009.

medical providers need to maintain a heightened level of SA. Combat conditions can yield a dynamic operational environment, in which tactical situations and missions can change suddenly. Should mass casualty circumstances emerge, it is essential for providers to stay alert to the mission, the current tactical situation, and the availability of medical resources. This triad of considerations may be less pressing when delivering care in garrison, but it must remain at the forefront of triage decisions when providing care to combat casualties.

Models for Analyzing Military Medical Support Postures

This report highlighted several modeling capabilities that can be applied to the problem sets that medical support personnel may face when grappling with the challenges outlined in the NDS. This appendix describes these models in more detail, including their use, their inputs, and the insights they can offer.

Prepositioning Requirements Planning Optimization

RAND researchers developed the Prepositioning Requirements Planning Optimization (PRePO) tool to integrate the numerous cost and logistics parameters and constraints related to warehousing. PRePO is designed to answer strategic-level questions about prepositioning WRM in theater. It computes the cost-optimal WRM posture to transport assets from storage sites in theater to their end-use locations. The core capability that shapes the prepositioning network is closure speed, or how quickly the assets must be moved. Due to the pivotal role this capability plays, closure time is the key driver behind system costs.[1]

---

[1] RAND previously developed a WRM optimization model known as the RAND Overseas Basing Optimization Tool. PRePO represents an evolution of this framework and extends the parameter and constraint sets of that earlier work. For more on the RAND Overseas Basing Optimization Tool, see Mahyar A. Amouzegar, Ronald G. McGarvey, Robert S. Tripp, Louis Luangkesorn, Thomas Lang, and Charles Robert Roll, Jr., *Evaluation of Options for Overseas Combat Support Basing*, Santa Monica, Calif.: RAND Corporation, MG-421-AF, 2006.

Inputs for Characterizing WRM Postures

PRePO requires a user to enter several input parameters, including

- the number, type, and physical characteristics of WRM assets to be stored
- characteristics of transportation modes, such as cargo capacities in terms of the size and weight of the cargo that each mode of transportation can carry, as well as the number of transports available within each mode type
- characteristics of facilities and points of end use, including storage facility location and square footage
- costs, such as the fixed costs for storing WRM at a facility (e.g., the annual cost for security contractors and support staff), a facility's marginal storage costs (e.g., the cost per square foot to lease warehouse space), and the maintenance cost for each type of WRM considered
- closure time, or the desired time frame within which the prepositioned WRM must be distributed to its points of end use.

Constraints for Bounding WRM Postures

The model must also ensure that an array of transportation and storage restrictions are satisfied. In so doing, PRePO emulates constraints that would exist in an actual warehousing and distribution network. These constraints fall into several categories:

- satisfy closure time limits
- respect facility capacity bounds
- honor vehicle capacity limits
- restrict vehicle throughput based on such considerations as berth capacity and other loading dock limitations
- manage fleet flow bounds, honoring vehicle utilization limits and fleet size restrictions.

PRePO WRM Assessments

After a run, PRePO generates the optimal prepositioning posture. It displays a record of which candidate storage facilities to use and how much of each type of WRM to assign to each storage facility. The model also displays a transportation network that indicates which storage locations serve each end-user location and how stored WRM is allocated to each end-user site. Using these results, PRePO generates a transportation schedule that indicates how WRM was allocated to vehicles via each modality, including the origin, destination, and time for each vehicle on that route. The final PRePO output is a set of costs, broken out into categories for facility operation, asset maintenance, asset storage, and transportation.

Blood Distribution Network Modeling

Building on the PRePO model, RAND researchers developed a dedicated tool to aid in the evaluation of theater-wide blood distribution networks. As noted earlier, blood support to combat operations poses an array of challenges further compounded by products with limited shelf lives that often require temperature controls during shipment. This can make for a difficult set of management decisions: How much of each blood product should be stored, and where, relative to the goal of meeting the needs of as many patients as possible?

Adding additional complications, the MHS offers a range of expeditionary capabilities for blood support. For example, specialty teams and kits can be deployed to collect blood from forces in the field. Transshipment teams can establish storage and distribution hubs in theater, receiving products from CONUS and routing them to destinations in theater. Red blood cells can be frozen, extending their shelf life of ten years—compared with only 21–42 days for liquid supplies, depending on the preservative solution used. The model accounts for these and other capabilities—for example, calculating the additional processing time before frozen cells can be used for a transfusion, as well as the specialized equipment required.

In the case of blood products, a key input to the optimization model is anticipated demand, by day and location. The model then evaluates where to deploy which expeditionary capabilities and in what amounts, as well as how much of each blood product to store at MTFs across the theater. In terms of constraints, the model honors the user's limits on local storage, bounds on the number and type of expeditionary capabilities that can be employed, and the availability of transport assets to move blood products from one node to another.

Medical Planners' Toolkit

MPTk, developed by the Naval Health Research Center, is a suite of databases and models designed to provide information on casualty distributions and the supply requirements for their care. It consists of four tools:[2]

- Patient condition occurrence frequencies. The user selects a historical contingency, choosing from a list of circumstances ranging from specific disaster response efforts to combat engagements. The tool then reports the frequency of injuries and illnesses over the course of that event.
- Casualty rate estimation. The user provides information related to the intensity level of an event—say, a force-on-force engagement. Drawing on data from a related injury distribution database, the tool reports the number, type, and timing of casualties stemming from a simulation of that event.
- Medical requirements estimation. Based on data from a user-run casualty estimation simulation, the tool generates reports on a range of medical supplies, equipment, and facilities used to treat casualties, assuming they are treated at a Role 3 medical facility. Outputs include the utilization of operating rooms and critical care wards, as well as key supplies, such as blood and blood products.
- Medical supply estimation. Narrower in focus than the previous tool, this package reports on a selected subset of consumable medical supplies. It then integrates these outputs into aggregate metrics, such as cost, weight, and the volume required for shipping.

---

[2] Naval Health Research Center, 2013b.

Joint Medical Planning Tool

JMPT, developed by the Naval Health Research Center and Teledyne Brown, is a stochastic simulation model designed to project medical outcomes over time stemming from the flow of casualties through a user-defined medical network.[3] The user can import a casualty distribution from a prior MPTk run or build a customized distribution based on injuries and diseases found in MPTk's patient condition database. The user then defines a treatment network, siting various medical provider roles using building blocks of capacity and capability that mirror existing expeditionary MHS facilities. The user can also input an evacuation network, specifying the number of evacuation vehicles and the routes they follow.

JMPT then simulates the flow of casualties through the network, reporting back such metrics as return-to-duty rates, the number of patients who died of their injuries, and the utilization of evacuation assets. The user has several options to conduct sensitivity analyses on those outcomes; JMPT allows the user to alter not only the network configuration and patient streams but also such factors as individual treatment facility capacities and the number of available medical providers in each facility.

---

[3]   Naval Health Research Center, "Joint Medical Planning Tool (JMPT): Medical Mission Support," San Diego, Calif., 2013a.

References

Air Force Pamphlet 10-1403, *Air Mobility Planning Factors*, Washington, D.C.: U.S. Department of the Air Force, October 24, 2018.

Air Force Tactics, Techniques, and Procedures 3-42.71, *Expeditionary Medical Support (EMEDS) and Air Force Theater Hospital (AFTH)*, Washington, D.C.: U.S. Department of the Air Force, August 27, 2014.

Ali, Idrees, and Phil Stewart, "More Than 100 U.S. Troops Diagnosed with Brain Injuries from Iran Attack," Reuters, February 10, 2020.

American Society of Health-System Pharmacists, "Drug Shortages Statistics," webpage, undated. As of December 9, 2020:
https://www.ashp.org/Drug-Shortages/Shortage-Resources/Drug-Shortages-Statistics

Amouzegar, Mahyar A., Ronald G. McGarvey, Robert S. Tripp, Louis Luangkesorn, Thomas Lang, and Charles Robert Roll, Jr., *Evaluation of Options for Overseas Combat Support Basing*, Santa Monica, Calif.: RAND Corporation, MG-421-AF, 2006. As of December 9, 2020:
https://www.rand.org/pubs/monographs/MG421.html

Amouzegar, Mahyar A., Robert S. Tripp, Ronald G. McGarvey, Edward W. Chan, and Charles Robert Roll, Jr., *Supporting Air and Space Expeditionary Forces: Analysis of Combat Support Basing Options*, Santa Monica, Calif.: RAND Corporation, MG-261-AF, 2004. As of December 9, 2020:
https://www.rand.org/pubs/monographs/MG261.html

Brennan, Zachary, "FDA Allows Temporary Saline Imports to Deal with Shortages Caused by Hurricane Maria," *Regulatory Focus*, October 11, 2017. As of December 9, 2020:
https://www.raps.org/regulatory-focus™/news-articles/2017/10/fda-allows-temporary-saline-imports-to-deal-with-shortages-caused-by-hurricane-maria

Brumfiel, Geoff, "Russia Seen Moving New Missiles to Eastern Europe," National Public Radio, December 8, 2016. As of December 9, 2020:
https://www.npr.org/sections/parallels/2016/12/08/504737811/russia-seen-moving-new-missiles-to-eastern-europe

Canadian North American Aerospace Defense Command Region Public Affairs, "Third Edition of the Arctic Air Power Seminar Welcomes International Experts Leaders, Military Members Alike," February 3, 2020. As of December 9, 2020: https://www.norad.mil/Francais/Article/2073332/third-edition-of-the-arctic-air-power-seminar-welcomes-international-experts-le

Castagna, Joanne, "Thule Air Base, Arctic—Consistently on Top of Its Game," U.S. Army, December 13, 2019. As of December 9, 2020: https://www.army.mil/article/230993/thule_air_base_arctic_consistently_on_top_of_its_game

Cavas, Christopher P., "CNO Bans 'A2AD' as Jargon," *Defense News*, October 3, 2016. As of December 9, 2020: https://www.defensenews.com/naval/2016/10/04/cno-bans-a2ad-as-jargon

Center for Strategic and International Studies, "Iranian Missile Launches: 1988–Present," *Missile Threat*, last updated February 10, 2020a. As of December 9, 2020: https://missilethreat.csis.org/iranian-missile-launches-1988-present

———, "Missiles of Russia," *Missile Threat*, last updated August 24, 2020b. As of December 9, 2020: https://missilethreat.csis.org/country/russia

———, "Missiles of North Korea," *Missile Threat*, last updated November 30, 2020c. As of December 9, 2020: https://missilethreat.csis.org/country/dprk

Chairman of the Joint Chiefs of Staff Instruction 4310.01E, *Logistics Planning Guidance for Pre-Positioned War Reserve Materiel*, Washington, D.C., January 13, 2020.

Coase, Ronald H., "The Nature of the Firm," *Economica*, Vol. 4, No. 16, November 1937, pp. 386–405.

Coram, Robert, *Boyd: The Fighter Pilot Who Changed the Art of War*, New York: Hachette Book Group, 2002.

Correll, John T., "Fighting Under Attack," *Air Force Magazine*, October 1, 1988. As of December 9, 2020: https://www.airforcemag.com/article/1088forward

Cowley, R. A., "A Total Emergency Medical System for the State of Maryland," *Maryland State Medical Journal*, Vol. 24, No. 7, July 1975, pp. 37–45.

Davis, Paul K., and Steven W. Popper, "Confronting Model Uncertainty in Policy Analysis for Complex Systems: What Policymakers Should Demand," *Journal on Policy and Complex Systems*, Vol. 5, No. 2, Fall 2019, pp. 181–201.

Defense and Veterans Brain Injury Center, "DoD Clinical Recommendation: Progressive Return to Activity Following Acute Concussion/Mild Traumatic Brain Injury: Guidance for the Primary Care Manager in Deployed and Non-Deployed Settings," Arlington, Va.: Defense Centers of Excellence for Psychological Health and Traumatic Brain Injury, January 2014.

Defense Health Agency, "DMLSS: Just-in-Time Logistics," factsheet, Falls Church, Va., February 2018.

———, "DCAM: Defense Medical Logistics Standard Support Customer Assistance Module," factsheet, Falls Church, Va., October 2020a.

———, "DML-ES/LogiCole: Innovative, Integrated, Intelligent," factsheet, Falls Church, Va., October 2020b.

———, "JMAR: Total Asset Medical Visibility," factsheet, Falls Church, Va., October 2020c.

———, "TEWLS: Modern Military Medical Logistics," factsheet, Falls Church, Va., October 2020d.

Densford, Fink, "Baxter Cleared from DoJ Antitrust Saline Probe," *Drug Delivery Business News*, February 1, 2019. As of August 3, 2020: https://www.drugdeliverybusiness.com/baxter-cleared-from-doj-antitrust-saline-probe

"A Dire Scarcity of Drugs Is Worsening, in Part, Because They Are So Cheap," *The Economist*, September 14, 2019.

Douglas, Jacob, "Zipline Testing Medical Supply Drones with US Military," CNBC, October 22, 2019. As of December 9, 2020: https://www.cnbc.com/2019/10/22/zipline-testing-medical-supply-drones-with-us-military.html

Drew, John G., Ronald G. McGarvey, and Peter Buryk, *Enabling Early Sustainment Decisions: Application to F-35 Depot-Level Maintenance*, Santa Monica, Calif.: RAND Corporation, RR-397-AF, 2013. As of December 9, 2020: https://www.rand.org/pubs/research_reports/RR397.html

Dupuy, Trevor N., *The Evolution of Weapons and Warfare*, Fairfax, Va.: Hero Books, 1984.

Erdbrink, Thomas, "Iran Reports Successful Launch of Missile as U.S. Considers New Sanctions," *New York Times*, July 27, 2017.

Executive Office of the President, *National Security Strategy of the United States of America*, Washington, D.C.: White House, December 2017.

Farmer, Carrie M., Heather Krull, Thomas W. Concannon, Molly M. Simmons, Francesca Pillemer, Teague Ruder, Andrew M. Parker, Maulik P. Purohit, Liisa Hiatt, Benjamin Saul Batorsky, and Kimberly A. Hepner, *Understanding Treatment of Mild Traumatic Brain Injury in the Military Health System*, Santa Monica, Calif.: RAND Corporation, RR-844-OSD, 2016. As of September 30, 2020:
https://www.rand.org/pubs/research_reports/RR844.html

Fazal, Tanisha M., Todd Rasmussen, Paul Nelson, and P. K. Carlton, "How Long Can the U.S. Military's Golden Hour Last?" *War on the Rocks*, October 8, 2018. As of December 9, 2020:
https://warontherocks.com/2018/10/how-long-can-the-u-s-military s-golden-hour-last

Fink, Sheri Lee, *War Hospital: A True Story of Surgery and Survival*, New York: Perseus Books, 2003.

———, *Five Days at Memorial: Life and Death in a Storm-Ravaged Hospital*, New York: Crown Publishers, 2013.

Gabriel, Richard A., and Karen S. Metz, *A History of Military Medicine*, 2 vols., New York: Greenwood Press, 1992.

Gilmore, Christopher K., Michael Chaykowsky, and Brent Thomas, *Autonomous Unmanned Aerial Vehicles for Blood Delivery: A UAV Fleet Design Tool and Case Study*, Santa Monica, Calif.: RAND Corporation, RR-3047-OSD, 2019. As of December 9, 2020:
https://www.rand.org/pubs/research_reports/RR3047.html

Goniewicz, Mariusz, "Effect of Military Conflicts on the Formation of Emergency Medical Services Systems Worldwide," *Academic Emergency Medicine*, Vol. 20, No. 5, May 2013, pp. 507–513.

Gormley, Dennis M., Andrew S. Erickson, and Jingdong Yuan, *A Low-Visibility Force Multiplier: Assessing China's Cruise Missile Ambitions*, Washington, D.C.: National Defense University Press, 2014.

Hamm, John A., *Improving the Air Force Medical Service's Expeditionary Medical Support System: A Simulation Approach: Analysis of Mass-Casualty Combat and Disaster Relief Scenarios*, dissertation, Santa Monica, Calif.: RAND Corporation, RGSD-A343-1, 2020. As of December 9, 2020:
https://www.rand.org/pubs/rgs_dissertations/RGSDA343-1.html

Heginbotham, Eric, Michael Nixon, Forrest E. Morgan, Jacob L. Heim, Jeff Hagen, Sheng Tao Li, Jeffrey Engstrom, Martin C. Libicki, Paul DeLuca, David A. Shlapak, David R. Frelinger, Burgess Laird, Kyle Brady, and Lyle J. Morris, *The U.S.-China Military Scorecard: Forces, Geography, and the Evolving Balance of Power, 1996–2017*, Santa Monica, Calif.: RAND Corporation, RR-392-AF, 2015. As of December 9, 2020:
https://www.rand.org/pubs/research_reports/RR392.html

Hlad, Jennifer, "Right Supplies, Right Place," *Air Force Magazine*, March 1, 2016.

Holcomb, John B., Lynn G. Stansbury, Howard R. Champion, Charles Wade, and Ronald F. Bellamy, "Understanding Combat Casualty Care Statistics," *Journal of Trauma*, Vol. 60, No. 2, February 2006, pp. 397–401.

ICU Medical, "Integrating ICU Medical Infusion Devices with Hospital EHR Decreased Major Dosing Errors by 52 Percent," press release, February 6, 2017. As of December 9, 2020:
https://www.icumed.com/about-us/news-events/news/2017/icu-medical-completes-the-acquisition-of-hospira-infusion-systems-from-pfizer

International Risk Governance Center, *Introduction to the IRGC Risk Governance Framework*, rev. ed., Lausanne, Switzerland, 2017.

"Iran Fires Long-Range Missiles into Indian Ocean in Military Drill—Media," Reuters, January 16, 2021.

"Iran—Strategic Weapon Systems," *Jane's Sentinel Security Assessment: The Gulf States*, page last updated November 1, 2020.

Ireland, John D., trans., *The Udana and the Itivuttaka: Two Classics from the Pali Canon*, Kandy, Sri Lanka: Buddhist Publication Society, 2007.

Irvani, Seyed M. R., "Design and Control Principles of Flexible Workforce in Manufacturing Systems," in James J. Cochran, Louis A. Cox, Jr., Pinar Keskinocak, Jeffrey P. Kharoufeh, and J. Cole Smith, eds., *Wiley Encyclopedia of Operations Research and Management Science*, Hoboken, N.J.: Wiley, 2011.

Iserson, Kenneth V., and John C. Moskop, "Triage in Medicine, Part I: Concept, History, and Types," *Annals of Emergency Medicine*, Vol. 49, No. 3, March 2007, pp. 275–281.

Jackson, F. Cameron, "Don't Get Wounded: Military Health System Consolidation and the Risk to Readiness," *Military Review*, September–October 2019, pp. 141–151.

Johnson, David E., and W. Bryan Gamble, "Trauma in the Arctic: An Incident Report," *Journal of Trauma*, Vol. 31, No. 10, October 1991, pp. 1340–1346.

Joint Publication 4-02, *Joint Health Services*, Washington, D.C.: U.S. Joint Chiefs of Staff, incorporating change 1, September 28, 2018.

Joint Publication 5-0, *Joint Planning*, Washington, D.C.: U.S. Joint Chiefs of Staff, June 16, 2017.

Kepe, Marta, "Lives on the Line: The A2AD Challenge to Combat Casualty Care," Modern War Institute at West Point, July 30, 2018. As of December 9, 2020:
https://mwi.usma.edu/lives-line-a2ad-challenge-combat-casualty-care

Kime, Patricia, "Services Turn Focus to Warfighters as DHA Takes over Military Hospitals," *Military.com*, April 3, 2019. As of December 9, 2020:
https://www.military.com/daily-news/2019/04/03/services-turn-focus-warfighter
s-dha-takes-over-military-hospitals.html

Kleiman, Michael P., "Global Patient Movement: Moving America's Ill and Injured Warfighters Safely, Securely, Soundly," U.S. Air Force, October 5, 2019. As of December 9, 2020:
https://www.af.mil/News/Article-Display/Article/1977765/global-patien
t-movement-moving-americas-ill-and-injured-warfighters-safely-secu

———, "U.S. Transportation Command Manages the Movement of America's Wounded Warfighters from Overseas to the Final Medical Treatment Destination Stateside," U.S. Air Force, January 8, 2020. As of December 9, 2020:
https://www.mcchord.af.mil/News/Article-Display/Article/2052474/
us-transportation-command-manages-the-movement-o
f-americas-wounded-warfighters/

Kovacs, Stephanie, Stephen E. Hawes, Stephen N. Maley, Emily Mosites, Ling Wong, and Andy Stergachis, "Technologies for Detecting Falsified and Substandard Drugs in Low and Middle-Income Countries," *PLoS One*, Vol. 9, No. 3, March 26, 2014, article e90601.

LaMattina, John, "Universities Stepping Up Efforts to Discover Drugs," *Forbes*, October 21, 2013.

Loftus, Peter, and Jonathan D. Rockoff, "Baxter Says Saline Shipments Disrupted in Hurricane-Wracked Puerto Rico," *Wall Street Journal*, September 27, 2017.

Lynch, Kristin F., Anthony DeCicco, Bart E. Bennett, John G. Drew, Amanda Kadlec, Vikram Kilambi, Kurt Klein, James A. Leftwich, Miriam E. Marlier, Ronald G. McGarvey, Patrick Mills, Theo Milonopoulos, Robert S. Tripp, and Anna Jean Wirth, *Analysis of Global Management of Air Force War Reserve Materiel to Support Operations in Contested and Degraded Environments*, Santa Monica, Calif., RAND Corporation, RR-3081-AF, 2021. As of March 22, 2021:
https://www.rand.org/pubs/research_reports/RR3081.html

Mayhew, Emily, *Wounded: A New History of the Western Front in World War I*, New York: Oxford University Press, 2014.

———, *A Heavy Reckoning: War, Medicine, and Survival in Afghanistan and Beyond*, London: Profile Books, 2017.

Mazer-Amirshahi, Maryann, and Erin R. Fox, "Saline Shortages—Many Causes, No Simple Solution," *New England Journal of Medicine*, Vol. 378, No. 16, April 19, 2018, pp. 1472–1474.

McGarvey, Ronald G., Manuel J. Carrillo, Douglas C. Cato, Jr., John G. Drew, Thomas Lang, Kristin F. Lynch, Amy L. Maletic, H. G. Massey, James M. Masters, Raymond A. Pyles, Ricardo Sanchez, Jerry M. Sollinger, Brent Thomas, Robert S. Tripp, and Ben D. Van Roo, *Analysis of the Air Force Logistics Enterprise: Evaluation of Global Repair Network Options for Supporting the F-16 and KC-135*, Santa Monica, Calif.: RAND Corporation, MG-872-AF, 2009. As of December 9, 2020:
https://www.rand.org/pubs/monographs/MG872.html

McGarvey, Ronald G., James M. Masters, Louis Luangkesorn, Stephen Sheehy, John G. Drew, Robert Kerchner, Ben D. Van Roo, and Charles Robert Roll, Jr., *Supporting Air and Space Expeditionary Forces: Analysis of CONUS Centralized Intermediate Repair Facilities*, Santa Monica, Calif.: RAND Corporation, MG-418-AF, 2008. As of December 9, 2020:
https://www.rand.org/pubs/monographs/MG418.html

McGarvey, Ronald G., Robert S. Tripp, Rachel Rue, Thomas Lang, Jerry M. Sollinger, Whitney A. Conner, and Louis Luangkesorn, *Global Combat Support Basing: Robust Prepositioning Strategies for Air Force War Reserve Materiel*, Santa Monica, Calif.: RAND Corporation, MG-902-AF, 2010. As of December 9, 2020:
https://www.rand.org/pubs/monographs/MG902.html

McKenna, Maryn, *Superbug: The Fatal Menace of MRSA*, New York: Free Press, 2010.

Military Health System, homepage, undated. As of July 16, 2020:
https://health.mil

———, "MHS Transformation," webpage, undated. As of December 9, 2020:
https://www.health.mil/Military-Health-Topics/MHS-Transformation

Moreno, J. Edward, "Kodak Wins $765M Federal Loan in Push to Produce Domestic Pharmaceuticals," *The Hill*, July 28, 2020. As of December 9, 2020:
https://thehill.com/homenews/administration/509330-kodak-wins-765m-federal-loan-in-push-to-produce-domestic

Moroney, Jennifer D. P., Stephanie Pezard, Laurel E. Miller, Jeffrey Engstrom, and Abby Doll, *Lessons from Department of Defense Disaster Relief Efforts in the Asia-Pacific Region*, Santa Monica, Calif.: RAND Corporation, RR-146-OSD, 2013. As of December 9, 2020:
https://www.rand.org/pubs/research_reports/RR146.html

Moshtaghian, Artemis, "Iran Launches Missiles into Eastern Syria, Targets ISIS," CNN, June 19, 2017. As of December 9, 2020:
https://www.cnn.com/2017/06/18/middleeast/iran-launches-missiles-into-syria

Moskop, John C., and Kenneth V. Iserson, "Triage in Medicine, Part II: Underlying Values and Principles," *Annals of Emergency Medicine*, Vol. 49, No. 3, March 2007, pp. 282–287.

Mouton, Christopher A., Edward W. Chan, Adam R. Grissom, John P. Godges, Badreddine Ahtchi, and Brian Dougherty, *Personnel Recovery in the AFRICOM Area of Responsibility: Cost-Effective Options for Improvement*, Santa Monica, Calif.: RAND Corporation, RR-2161/1-AFRICOM, 2019. As of December 9, 2020: https://www.rand.org/pubs/research_reports/RR2161z1.html

Naval Health Research Center, "Joint Medical Planning Tool (JMPT): Medical Mission Support," San Diego, Calif., 2013a. As of December 9, 2020: https://www.med.navy.mil/sites/nmrc/nhrc/Documents/jmpt_2013.pdf

———, "Medical Planners' Toolkit (MPTk): Medical Mission Support," San Diego, Calif., 2013b. As of December 9, 2020: https://www.med.navy.mil/sites/nmrc/nhrc/Documents/MPTk_2013.pdf

Office of the Under Secretary of Defense for Policy, *Report to Congress: Department of Defense Arctic Strategy*, Washington, D.C., June 2019.

O'Mahony, Angela, Ilana Blum, Gabriela Armenta, Nicholas Burger, Joshua Mendelsohn, Michael J. McNerney, Steven W. Popper, Jefferson P. Marquis, and Thomas S. Szayna, *Assessing, Monitoring, and Evaluating Army Security Cooperation: A Framework for Implementation*, Santa Monica, Calif.: RAND Corporation, RR-2165-A, 2018. As of December 9, 2020: https://www.rand.org/pubs/research_reports/RR2165.html

Oswald, Kirsty, "US$1 Test Card Can Detect Poor Quality Ceftriaxone Antibiotic," *Pharmaceutical Journal*, August 31, 2016.

Palmer, Eric, "Pfizer Subpoenaed to Testify in DOJ's Antitrust Probe of Saline Shortages," *Fierce Pharma*, April 20, 2017a. As of December 9, 2020: https://www.fiercepharma.com/legal/pfizer-subpoenaed-to-testify-doj-s-antitrust-probe-saline-shortages

———, "Baxter Expects $70M Sales Hit from Hurricane Damage; Amgen Says Costs Could Top $165M," *Fierce Pharma*, October 25, 2017b. As of December 9, 2020: https://www.fiercepharma.com/pharma/baxter-expects-70-million-sales-hit-from-hurricane-damage

Pandolf, Kent B., and Robert E. Burr, eds., *Medical Aspects of Harsh Environments*, Falls Church, Va.: U.S. Army Office of the Surgeon General, 2001.

Parsons, Patrick B., *Medical Support for Combat Operations in a Denied Environment (MS-CODE): Considerations for Immediate and Future Operations and Research Across the Strategic, Operational, and Tactical Domains*, Maxwell Air Force Base: Air War College, April 6, 2017.

Paul, Christopher, Michael Nixon, Heather Peterson, Beth Grill, and Jessica Yeats, *The RAND Security Cooperation Prioritization and Propensity Matching Tool*, Santa Monica, Calif.: RAND Corporation, TL-112-OSD, 2013. As of December 9, 2020: https://www.rand.org/pubs/tools/TL112.html

Payne, Craig, *Principles of Naval Weapons System*s, 2nd ed., Annapolis, Md.: Naval Institute Press, 2010.

Philpott, Tom, "More Than 17,000 Uniformed Medical Jobs Eyed for Elimination," *Military.com*, January 10, 2019. As of December 9, 2020: https://www.military.com/daily-news/2019/01/10/more-17000-uniformed-medical-jobs-eyed-elimination.html

Public Law 116–92, National Defense Authorization Act for Fiscal Year 2020, December 20, 2019.

"Qatar Airways Threatens to Sue over 'Illegal' Gulf Blockade," Al Jazeera, July 15, 2020.

Rabin, Roni Caryn, "Why Lifesaving Drugs May Be Missing on Your Next Flight," *New York Times*, October 3, 2019.

Rawls, John, *A Theory of Justice*, Cambridge, Mass.: Harvard University Press, 1971.

Raymond, Nate, "U.S. Closes IV Solution Shortage Antitrust Probe, Baxter Says," Reuters, February 22, 2019.

Resnick, Adam C., Kathryn Connor, Anna Jean Wirth, and Eric DuBois, *Optimizing Army Medical Materiel Strategy*, Santa Monica, Calif.: RAND Corporation, RR-2646-A, 2019. As of December 9, 2020: https://www.rand.org/pubs/research_reports/RR2646.html

Roblin, Sebastien, "Will Blood-Bearing Delivery Drones Transform Disaster Relief and Battlefield Medicine?" *Forbes*, October 22, 2019.

Rostker, Bernard D., *Providing for the Casualties of War: The American Experience Through World War II*, Santa Monica, Calif.: RAND Corporation, MG-1164-OSD, 2013. As of December 9, 2020: https://www.rand.org/pubs/monographs/MG1164.html

Rostker, Bernard D., Charles Nemfakos, Henry A. Leonard, Elliot Axelband, Abby Doll, Kimberly N. Hale, Brian McInnis, Richard Mesic, Daniel Tremblay, Roland J. Yardley, and Stephanie Young, *Building Toward an Unmanned Aircraft System Training Strategy*, Santa Monica, Calif.: RAND Corporation, RR-440-OSD, 2014. As of December 9, 2020: https://www.rand.org/pubs/research_reports/RR440.html

"Russian Federation—Strategic Weapon Systems," *Jane's Sentinel Security Assessment: Russia and the CIS*, last updated April 16, 2020.

Sack, Thomas L., "Improved Combat Casualty Medicine," *Air Force Magazine*, August 1, 1981. As of December 9, 2020: https://www.airforcemag.com/article/0881medicine

Schanz, Marc V., "Infrastructure Improvements Key to Engagement," *Air Force Magazine*, July 9, 2015.

———, "Hardening, Dispersal, and Survivability in Europe," *Air Force Magazine*, September 15, 2015.

Simchi-Levi, David, *Operations Rules: Delivering Customer Value Through Flexible Operations*, Cambridge, Mass.: MIT Press, 2010.

Snyder, Don, Edward W. Chan, James J. Burks, Mahyar A. Amouzegar, and Adam C. Resnick, *How Should Air Force Expeditionary Medical Capabilities Be Expressed?* Santa Monica, Calif.: RAND Corporation, MG-785-AF, 2009. As of December 9, 2020:
https://www.rand.org/pubs/monographs/MG785.html

Sternberg, Steve, "A Crack in the Armor: Military Health System Isn't Ready for Battlefield Injuries," *U.S. News and World Report*, October 10, 2019. As of December 9, 2020:
https://www.usnews.com/news/national-news/articles/2019-10-10/military-health-system-isnt-ready-for-battlefield-injuries

Swaminathan, Jayashankar M., "Enabling Customization Using Standardized Operations," *California Management Review*, Vol. 43, No. 3, Spring 2001, pp. 125–135.

Thomas, Brent, Mahyar A. Amouzegar, Rachel Costello, Robert A. Guffey, Andrew Karode, Christopher Lynch, Kristin F. Lynch, Ken Munson, Chad J. R. Ohlandt, Daniel M. Romano, Ricardo Sanchez, Robert S. Tripp, and Joseph V. Vesely, *Project AIR FORCE Modeling Capabilities for Support of Combat Operations in Denied Environments*, Santa Monica, Calif., RAND Corporation, RR-427-AF, 2015. As of December 9, 2020:
http://www.rand.org/pubs/research_reports/RR427.html

Thomas, Brent, Katherine Anania, Anthony DeCicco, and John A. Hamm, *Toward Resiliency in the Joint Blood Supply Chain*, Santa Monica, Calif.: RAND Corporation, RR-2482-DARPA, 2018. As of December 9, 2020:
https://www.rand.org/pubs/research_reports/RR2482.html

Tingstad, Abbie, *Climate Change and U.S. Security in the Arctic*, testimony presented to the Subcommittee on Transportation and Maritime Security, Committee on Homeland Security, U.S. House of Representatives, Santa Monica, Calif.: RAND Corporation, CT-517, September 19, 2019. As of December 9, 2020:
https://www.rand.org/pubs/testimonies/CT517.html

Tingstad, Abbie, Stephanie Pezard, and Scott Stephenson, "Will the Breakdown in U.S.-Russia Cooperation Reach the Arctic?" *Inside Sources*, October 12, 2016. As of December 9, 2020:
https://www.insidesources.com/will-the-breakdown-in-u-s-russia-cooperation-reach-the-arctic

Tweh, Bowdeya, "Justice Department Investigating Baxter Over Saline Shortage," *Wall Street Journal*, May 5, 2017.

Upton, David M., "The Management of Manufacturing Flexibility," *California Management Review*, Vol. 36, No. 2, 1994, pp. 72–89.

U.S. Army Office of the Surgeon General, *Emergency War Surgery*, 5th rev. ed., Fort Sam Houston, Tex., 2018.

U.S. Code, Title 10, Armed Forces, Section 1073c, Administration of Defense Health Agency and Military Medical Treatment Facilities.

U.S. Department of the Air Force, *Arctic Strategy: Ensuring a Stable Arctic Through Vigilance, Power Projection, Cooperation, and Preparation*, Washington, D.C., July 21, 2020.

U.S. Department of Defense, *Report on the Status of Department of Defense Programs for Prepositioning of Materiel and Equipment*, Washington, D.C., 2014.

———, *Summary of the 2018 National Defense Strategy of the United States of America: Sharpening the American Military's Competitive Edge*, Washington, D.C., 2018.

U.S. Food and Drug Administration, "FDA Drug Shortages: Current and Resolved Drug Shortages and Discontinuations Reported to FDA," data set, undated. As of December 9, 2020:
https://www.accessdata.fda.gov/scripts/drugshortages/default.cfm

U.S. House of Representatives, Committee on Energy and Commerce, Subcommittee on Oversight and Investigation, "The Heparin Disaster: Chinese Counterfeits and American Failures," hearing transcript, Washington, D.C., April 29, 2008.

U.S. Marine Corps, *Marine Corps Class VIIIA Handbook*, Washington, D.C., NAVMC 4000.2A, June 23, 2017.

U.S. Pacific Command, "Improving Disaster Response Through a Reliable Blood Supply," April 21, 2015. As of December 9, 2020:
https://www.pacom.mil/Media/News/Article/586171/improving-disaster-response-through-a-reliable-blood-supply

Wendelbo, Morten, and Christine Crudo Blackburn, "A Saline Shortage This Flu Season Exposes a Flaw in Our Medical Supply Chain," *Smithsonian Magazine*, January 22, 2018. As of February 3, 2020:
https://www.smithsonianmag.com/innovation/saline-shortage-this-flu-season-exposes-flaw-in-our-medical-supply-chain-180967879

White, Douglas B., Mitchell H. Katz, John M. Luce, and Bernard Lo, "Who Should Receive Life Support During a Public Health Emergency? Using Ethical Principles to Improve Allocation Decisions," *Annals of Internal Medicine*, Vol. 150, No. 2, January 20, 2009, pp. 132–138.

White, Melissa B., "Natural Disaster Response Improved at Cope North 15," U.S. Air Force, February 23, 2015. As of December 9, 2020:
http://www.af.mil/News/ArticleDisplay/tabid/223/Article/566834

Whitesides, George M., "The Origins and the Future of Microfluidics," *Nature*, Vol. 442, No. 7107, July 27, 2006, pp. 368–373.

Yeebo, Yepoka, "The African Startup Using Phones to Spot Counterfeit Drugs," *Bloomberg Businessweek*, July 31, 2015.

Zaman, Muhammad H., *Bitter Pills: The Global War on Counterfeit Drugs*, New York: Oxford University Press, 2018.